PUBLIC RELATIONS
FOR
NURSING HOMES

PUBLIC RELATIONS
—FOR—
NURSING HOMES

By

JOHN PHILIP BACHNER

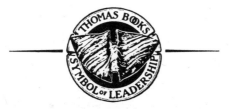

CHARLES C THOMAS • PUBLISHER
Springfield • Illinois • U.S.A.

Published and Distributed Throughout the World by

CHARLES C THOMAS • PUBLISHER

Bannerstone House

301-327 East Lawrence Avenue, Springfield, Illinois, U.S.A.

© *1974, by* CHARLES C THOMAS • PUBLISHER

ISBN 0-398-03111-8

Library of Congress Catalog Card Number: 73 23027

*With THOMAS BOOKS careful attention is given to all details of
manufacturing and design. It is the Publisher's desire to present books that
are satisfactory as to their physical qualities and artistic possibilities and
appropriate for their particular use. THOMAS BOOKS will be true to those
laws of quality that assure a good name and good will.*

Printed in the United States of America

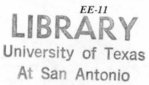
Library of Congress Cataloging in Publication Data

Bachner, John Philip.
    Public relations for nursing homes.

    1. Public relations—Nursing homes. I. Title.
[DNLM: 1. Hospital administration   2. Nursing homes   3. Public
relations. WX150 B124p 1974]
RA997.B28   659.2′9′36216   73–23027
ISBN 0–398–03111–8

For My Mother

For A Thousand Different Reasons

CONTENTS

Part II

Public and Relations

PREFACE

THERE IS NO MYSTERY to public relations. It involves a variety of practices and skills which, for the most part, can be carried out adequately by any person possessing average intelligence, common sense, and basic instructions, such as those presented in this book.

Because you are reading this book, it is fair to assume that you are at least mildly interested in the subject of public relations. But you may be in for a difficult time unless you are prepared to shed some preconceived notions about PR and see it primarily as the art of communicating truth.

To begin with, public relations can be defined no more precisely than by saying it is the art of communicating to your publics—publics, plural, because there are many identifiable groups (such as patients, patients' families, visitors, employees, etc.) with whom you are concerned.

Communication is not a self-understood word. One communicates in ways far beyond the written or spoken word. More specifically, communication occurs whenever matter transmitted impinges on a sense and is given to the brain for analysis and interpretation. For example, if you enter the home of a friend and smell mouth-watering aromas emanating from the kitchen, chances are you will think your friend's wife is a good cook. Why? Because the odor which impinged upon the sense of smell was analyzed and interpreted by the brain. If you sit down to dinner, however, and the food is absolutely terrible, the sense of taste will lead to the decision that the wife, after all, may not be such a good cook. In other words, any one of the five senses can be used to receive communicated matter, whether it was communicated intentionally or not, even though eyes and ears usually are the most commonly used receptors. The analysis which the brain turns out, sometimes in conjunction with the imagination, is termed an image. The extent of the image depends on the extent of communication. Going back to our previous example, if you never met the friend's wife, but only tasted the food, your only image of her probably would be that of a bad cook. But since you probably will chat with her, you will be able to develop a more complete image, which includes "bad cook" as a portion.

Unfortunately, with the hectic pace of today's world, most people do not communicate with others to a degree sufficient to produce a rounded image. As a result, the image generated within a given context often serves as the image of the whole person.

For example, an employee usually sees you in one light only, as the boss. If he were asked how you are as a family man, he probably would base his opinion on his image of you as his employer. Similarly, if a prospective patient's family finds you to be very busy and unable to give them the time they feel they deserve, they probably will develop an image of you as "too involved with administrative affairs to be concerned with personalities." *This image of you then will serve as the image they have of the nursing home,* perhaps conceiving it as callous; not really concerned with the patients. In other words, just as one small encounter can serve as the basis for an image of a whole person, so can the image of a person serve as the basis for an image of whomever or whatever that person represents. Of course, the image developed may be entirely false. But that is not the point. The point is that an image will be formed regardless. And here is where public relations comes in.

One of the main purposes of public relations is to control projection of an image to as great an extent as possible, so you can control to as great a degree as possible what others think of you and what you represent. In this regard, there are two important considerations.

First, it is imperative that the correct information is communicated to the public involved. Every person, every facility, is multifaceted. To try to convey all facts of a personality is impossible. Therefore, when communicating, it is imperative that it first be determined what the public most wants to know about, and then communicate it. For example, given limited time, a prospective patient's family wants to know about what care the patient will receive and related factors. To go into a discussion of employee benefits would be foolhardy. Therefore, when developing an image, one must adjust image forming material to the situation at hand and the public involved.

Second, the image must be truthful. It is a relatively simple matter to generate a false image. It involves creation of programs which promote half-truths or omit critical information. But is it worth it? When people realize that an image is false, they to an extent perceive the person possessing the image as a liar, someone who has raised the level of expectation, thereby making the fall to truth that much more painful. Going back to the cooking example, if the friend built up an image of his wife as a superlative cook, you would be very disappointed when the meal turned out poorly. Conversely, if no mention was made of her cooking ability, you would be disappointed, but not nearly as disappointed as if you had been looking forward to a gourmet delight.

So much for theory. The balance of this book discusses actual programs to which you should give serious consideration. For the most part they cost very little. In many cases they cost nothing. Nor are they designed to create a good image of the home purely for the sake of having a good image. They are designed to assist in keeping down the vacancy rate, keeping down employee turnover and, in general, to provide tangible, practical benefits whose value far exceeds the investment made.

PUBLIC RELATIONS
FOR
NURSING HOMES

PART I

PUBLIC RELATIONS
TOOLS AND TECHNIQUES

I

DEVELOPING A
PUBLIC RELATIONS PROGRAM

BEFORE YOU CAN do anything in terms of Public Relations (PR) programming, you first must be somewhat familiar with the various tools and techniques of PR, the current state of relations with your various publics, what needs to be done, and the resources available to you.

Guidance Materials

Guidance materials are those instructional publications which will provide you with some basic information on public relations. It is our obviously biased opinion that this book provides you with a comprehensive amount of guidance material which heretofore was unavailable between two covers and, in some cases, just unavailable. This is not to say that you should not look at other PR materials. No source can tell you everything, and only through absorbing as much material as possible can you get the ideas or germs of ideas required to develop and conduct an excellent program.

The PR Audit

The PR audit is a relatively uncomplicated program which goes a long way toward helping you establish your program. A few guidelines are discussed below.

BE FAMILIAR WITH GUIDANCE MATERIAL. We suggest that you read both parts of this book to get a feel for PR. You may wish to take notes, dog-ear or underline as you go along for reference later.

DETERMINE WHO YOUR PUBLICS ARE. Determine who your publics are by using PART II of the book as a basic guide. It is suggested that you break any general public (such as employees) into as many different subpublics as possible (nursing personnel, dietary personnel, etc.), as it is far easier to consider a public in terms of several manageable units, rather than one large one.

5

DETERMINE WHAT YOU HAVE BEEN AND ARE DOING. For each public and/or subpublic list exactly what you have done or are doing in terms of communicating and public relations, including the tools you use for implementation purposes.

DETERMINE RESOURCES. Determine what resources are available to you, including in-house equipment which you can employ in a PR program; personnel whose talents could be used, and, of course, budget.

RANK BY IMPORTANCE AND NEEDS. To the best of your ability, rank each public and subpublic in terms of its importance to you. Determine where immediate action is necessary by correlating importance of the public with amount of activity devoted to it. For example, if relations with the #1 public are fair to somewhat adequate, but relations with the #2 public are poor, #2 is your immediate concern.

ESTABLISH GOALS AND STRATEGIES. Establishment of goals in terms of publics with which you want to improve relations and strategies (the means by which you will achieve the goals) are a direct outgrowth of the PR audit. In essence, they are the backbone of your PR program and should be formulated in terms of general PR programs and tools and the specific conditions which prevail. Use the index of this book for cross reference purposes, and do not be afraid to modify, disregard or invent. In all cases, keep track of what you are doing. Attempt to get as much feedback as possible. Put the greatest effort into programs which will yield the best results. Above all, be honest—with yourself and others. If what you have to say and show is truthful, you have half the battle won, and your PR effort will have to be geared only to making others believe.

II

PHYSICAL PLANT
EVALUATION

Visual communication is the means by which your nursing home communicates most frequently to most publics. In fact, it probably is not unfair to state that most people in your community know of your home's existence only because they have driven or walked by it. If the paint is peeling; if a window or two is broken; if the home and grounds in any way look less than appealing and clean, you are doing untold harm to your image. Those who see the exterior in a state of disrepair immediately will assume that the interior is in similar condition and that management and staff most probably have a careless attitude about their own appearance and responsibilities. On the other hand, if your home is in a good state of repair; if the grounds are well-planted and well-maintained, those who see it assume that it is just as attractive inside and that management and staff most likely have pride in the facility and the manner in which they provide care for their patients. Old adages not withstanding, books frequently are judged by their cover and, unless read, the judgment stands as truth.

Exterior Appearance Evaluation Program

Obviously, it is to your benefit to ensure that your nursing home has as attractive an exterior appearance as possible. It is suggested that a thorough independent evaluation be made by someone not involved directly with the nursing home, possibly a friend or acquaintance. In asking for an evaluation, be sure to express your desire for absolutely frank comments, the more critical the better. Also consider evaluating the street on which the home is located. If conditions warrant, contact local government officials regarding neighborhood improvement programs. After all, the value of your nursing home, and the image people have of it, are

very much affected by the condition of its immediate environment. If the neighborhood is beginning to go downhill, it will
take your nursing home with it.

Once an initial evaluation of the home is made, you should
make it a point to inspect the home, grounds and neighborhood
as frequently as once a month, as objectively as possible, to ensure
that the visual image your home projects is as favorable as possible.

Interior Evaluation Program

The evaluation of the sensual impact of your home's interior is
far more involved than that of exterior. Items to consider are,
among others:

CLEANLINESS OF FACILITY. Floors, walls, ceilings, furnishings, etc., must
be kept clean and in a state of good repair.

DECORATIONS. The home's appearance should be somewhat lively and
colorful, appearing more like a community and a home than just a
drab health care facility. There should be graphics and other framed
materials on the walls, such as paintings, photographs, diplomas, certificates of inspection, etc., which must be hung straight and framed
well. To display a license that is poorly framed and dusty indicates
that it isn't very important to you.

PERSONNEL. Since an evaluation of the quality of care provided very
often is made on the basis of how personnel look and act, be certain
that they dress correctly and carry themselves properly in their relations with patients, fellow employees, visitors and others.

PATIENTS. Patients should be involved and active, not simply sitting
around all day and staring at a flickering television. If the latter is
true, regardless of what the facts of the matter are, it indicates that patients are not involved in activities, nor in life itself.

The list, of course, is endless. A program of evaluation involves
nothing more than keeping your senses alert as you move through
your nursing home, trying to evaluate what you see, hear, smell,
touch and taste as objectively as possible.

One excellent means for evaluating your home objectively is to
utilize materials on selection of a nursing home available from
various associations and the government. One such publication is
Nursing Home Care, stock number 1761–00032, Superintendent
of Documents, U.S. Government Printing Office, Washington,

D.C. 20402. Price is 45 cents. In it is a lengthy checklist which "consumers" are supposed to use in evaluating a nursing home. Use it on your own home to determine how you rate.

III

PRINTED MATERIAL

A NY PIECE OF printed material bearing the name of your nursing home represents your nursing home. To a very real extent, any letter sent on your letterhead in your envelope is an ambassador. If the letterhead is well-designed and attractive, it indicates concern about details and depth of professionalism. Conversely, a cluttered, poorly designed letterhead can have a decidedly negative effect, a risk hardly worth assuming when one realizes that there is little cost difference between material which conveys a positive image and that which detracts from it.

Analyze Your Home's Printed Material

To determine the image value of your home's printed material, gather together a sample of everything which bears its name. Divide material into two groups: external material, that which usually is sent to those outside the home, such as letterheads, second sheets, envelopes, business cards and billing forms, and internal material, used primarily for in-house communication, including staff memoranda forms, newsletters, bulletins, and so forth.

All printed material, and especially external material, should be carefully and critically examined, preferably by someone capable of objectivity, and aware of what works well and what does not. For example, a well-designed letterhead is simple and uncluttered, conveying the image of the home. If the image is modern, then modern design is employed; if the image is traditional, then traditional design is used, often as a function of the type face selected.

In addition, all external material should appear to come from the same design and paper family, although different paper weights will be involved, business card paper being heavier than letterhead paper, for example. By standardizing in this manner, you gain even more control over the image conveyed.

If your home's external material is in need of improvement; if the letterhead is cluttered; if design changes from business card to envelope; if different colors or types of paper are utilized, then it is time for a new, standardized design.

Obtaining New Material

To make an investment in new printed materials worthwhile, obtain professional assistance, either from a competent public relations, advertising or commercial art firm or, at a lesser rate, from free-lance talent, or the art staff of a printing firm. In all cases, ask to see samples of work before making a selection.

The first step usually is to concentrate on the design of the letterhead. Do not be afraid to include information which you feel is important, such as memberships in well-known national associations or programs for which the home is qualified. This material usually can be included in a very neat, uncluttered manner. By the same token, do not overdo it, and do not include references to organizations to which membership is not continuous.

The graphic designer should be able to present at least several different designs for you to choose from. Once you do make a selection, it will be the design basis for other material, such as second sheet, business cards, etc.

Once design is determined, the designer should be able to provide assistance in determining the color of the paper to be used as well as the color of the ink. While using corrective fluid on colored stock used to be impossible, it no longer is, in that color-matched corrective fluid can be obtained from firms such as Liquid Paper, usually available through an office supply establishment.

In-house material of course does not have to be as well done as that used for out-of-home communication. Nonetheless, you may find that, even though less expensive paper is used, the same graphic designs can be utilized. If you are willing to undertake the additional expense, it would be to your good to have all printed materials professionally designed to accurately portray your image to all who come into contact with it.

IV

IDEA NOTEBOOK

PERHAPS ONE OF the most important of all tools for anyone involved in public relations is a small pocket notebook used for jotting down ideas. First, it allows you to jot down an idea immediately (an excellent habit to get into) and, second, it allows you to keep a central location for ideas, rather than scattering them about. Suggested for use is a small spiral-bound notebook about two inches by four inches which allows you to place a small pen securely in the spiral binding. Alternatives to consider are tape recorders and dictating devices, some of which are made specifically for noting of ideas.

Remember, ideas are precious things and often fleeting. Don't trust to a crowded memory what can easily be secured for future use.

V

WRITING

WRITING IS AN ESSENTIAL element of any public relations/
communications program. It is utilized in development of
memoranda, bulletins, brochures, news releases, speeches, letters-
to-the-editor, day-to-day correspondence and in countless other
ways.

There are several methods available for establishing an other-
than-routine writing capability for your nursing home. You can
do it yourself, have someone on staff do it for you, or utilize free-
lance talent or a PR firm to edit or prepare all copy. Regardless
of budget or other circumstances, it is advisable to hire professional assistance at least for the most important projects, such as
a brochure, which will be read by hundreds of different people.
To undertake such a project on your own is to risk putting into
print an inadvertent misstatement which could make the brochure
at best counterproductive.

Doing It Yourself

Assuming for the time being that most writing will not involve
special projects, here follow some basic guidelines to help ensure
that whatever you write—be it a memo or magazine article—says
exactly what you want it to say.

1. KNOW YOUR SUBJECT. Know exactly what you want or are supposed
to write about. Don't just "feel confident." Be positive. In this way you
will minimize chances that you will roam from the core of the matter.
You will not have to include confusing, extraneous material because
"maybe it should be included." In fact, it often is valuable to write
the exact subject on a piece of paper to be kept in sight at all times.

2. DETERMINE RESEARCH REQUIREMENTS. By knowing exactly what your
subject is, you know exactly what topics require research or the back-
ing of statistics and data. Much of what you need probably is available
from a library; from your own files, or from national associations.
Where necessary, arrange for interviews to supplement written research
materials.

3. READ ALL RESEARCH MATERIAL AT LEAST TWICE. Your first reading

of research material should give you a general grasp of how things fit together. Take notes as you read, indicating in them the source of the note, including title and page number. Once done, reread research material in light of your general, overall grasp of the subject, taking more notes and jotting down ideas on how to use the material, how it correlates with other research, etc. You may wish to take notes on 3 x 5 cards on the first reading; reassemble into logical order, and schedule rereading of research materials based on the logical order.

4. MAKE REFLECTIVE NOTES. Once you've read your research material at least twice, think about what you've read while reviewing whatever notes you've taken. Whatever relevant thoughts come to mind should be noted, regardless of whether or not you think they will be used. Remember: You can always delete words and ideas while in the writing stage, while nothing is more disheartening than reading your published work only to see that something has been left out.

5. CATEGORIZE. Take a long hard look at all your notes and ideas. Categorize them under subject or topic headings, each section being an overall element of the entire piece. If you feel that a certain item is a subcategory, label it as such.

6. OUTLINE. Examine your subject headings and determine in what order they should flow. If you're dealing in terms of chronology, the task is simple. More often than not, however, you will be dealing with ideas, which necessitates the most important event or idea coming first, with each succeeding topic being related to the one which preceded it.

7. TALK OR WRITE IT THROUGH. Working with your outline, talk your story through as if you were writing it. You should be able to go in a straight line, from Point A to Point B to Point C, etc., without having to explain some aspect of Point A in the middle of Point C. If you do, something is wrong and it probably will be best for you to change your outline to accommodate a smooth flow of ideas. If you can type or write rapidly, and prefer either method to "talking it through," use it providing you will not become wedded to your output. The sole purpose of this exercise is to generate thought and see if the outline will work.

8. START WRITING. Begin writing by working with your outline and bringing in all the facts, names, dates, and other material which are even remotely relevant. Don't worry about grammar and style. Worry only about getting down all your thoughts and all back-up material.

9. DOUBLE CHECK CONTENTS AND ORGANIZATION. Read what you have written and answer the following three questions as critically as possible: Have I included everything I possibly can? Is everything I've said nonrepetitious and absolutely relevant and essential? Do my thoughts follow one another in a smooth-flowing, logical order? Add,

delete, rewrite and reorganize (with scissors and cellophane tape, if necessary) until you can answer the three questions with a "yes."

10. PERFORM PRELIMINARY (ROUGH) EDITING. Check what you have written for correct grammar, spelling, statistical recording, and so forth.

11. PERFORM MAJOR EDITING. Go through the rough-edited text to ensure that you have said everything as simply and clearly as possible. Rambling, run-on sentences should be broken into shorter ones. Check relative pronouns (like which, what, who, etc.) to be sure that it is clear to whom or to what they refer. Where possible, make a passive voice active, e.g., "she did" rather than "it was done by her." Avoid pejoratives (words which indicate a bias,) such as "only six," where the "only" indicates that, in the writer's mind, it was not enough. Use the simplest word possible, unless no other word will do (such as "pejorative,") and be sure to explain words which may not be understood readily. Remember: If you have to use a hypothetical example to illustrate a word it may mean that you did not do a good enough job of explaining what the word really means.

12. WRITE/REWRITE INTRODUCTION AND CONCLUSION. The purpose of an introduction is to tell the reader what you are about to tell him. The conclusion or summary more or less tells him what you've just told him. In both cases, it's easier to write these sections once you've done the "telling" and, in some cases, you may find that writing and rewriting leads you to conclusions different from those first anticipated.

13. SUBMIT TO DEVIL'S ADVOCATES. Once you have the piece in what you feel to be finished form, submit a copy to two persons, one familiar with the subject matter who should be asked to comment on content, the other unfamiliar with subject matter who should be asked to comment on the way you've said what you've said. Encourage written comments on each copy.

14. CONSIDER COMMENTS BEFORE REWRITING. Consider all comments carefully before rewriting. If a major item of content is debatable, seek another opinion. If several people concur that something is wrong, by all means rewrite, even major sections. Pay particular attention to the comments of the person unfamiliar with subject matter. If he became confused, you're not communicating well enough and more work is needed.

Obtaining Outside Talent

In some cases you may wish to have a piece written totally by or at least edited by free-lance or full-time professional writing talent. Several sources for such assistance are available. Perhaps the best source is a local newspaper. Determine the name of one or two writers by checking bylines. Call the paper and speak with the writer. Ask him if he does free-lance work. Chances are he will. It should be noted that the newspaper is an excellent source not only because of available writing talent, but also because it gives you a contact at the local newspaper. Other sources are: Yellow Pages (under "writers"), classified section of a local newspaper (under "personal services"), or a journalism professor or instructor from a nearby college or university. In hiring a free-lance writer, expect to pay between $10 and $15 per hour, based on the experience and qualifications of the individual involved. For best results, give him at least a rough outline of the ideas you wish covered. This will save time going back and forth.

To select a public relations firm, follow those selection guidelines given in Chapter XX which relate to advertising firms.

VI

INTERPERSONAL
COMMUNICATIONS

IN MANY INSTANCES, a public or subpublic of a public relations
program can involve just one person, as representative of a public or as an individual member of a public. In such cases, planning
entails several considerations. One consideration is image control.
While you want to relate those elements of yourself, your nursing
home program, or what have you which best coincide with the
interest of the public concerned, you also want to relate them in a
way which best corresponds to the public's interests. Similarly,
when you wish an action from the public, it most often is the way
in which you make the action request which will determine
whether or not the desired action is performed.

On a one-to-one basis, interpersonal communications involves,
more than anything else, empathy—the ability to place yourself in
someone else's shoes.

For example, assuming the public is the son of a patient who
has claimed bitterly, and totally without foundation in fact, that
staff has been callous, food terrible, etc. The son calls you and is
understandably angry. If you merely state over the phone that the
story is untrue, and merely a typical reaction of a newly-arrived
patient trying to stir up guilt feelings in the son, you probably
will get nowhere. Understanding the person's frame of mind,
therefore, it is best to invite him to the nursing home at any time
to see for himself that the story is without foundation. And if he
is concerned enough to make the trip, by all means show him
around, let him see what really goes on, and perhaps give him
advice on interpersonal communication vis-a-vis his relationship
with the patient. In other words, you first must recognize his
frame of mind and his concern, and develop the appropriate response.

Similarly, when motivation is involved, we can take the example of a reasonably good employee who for some reason is not performing well on the job. Your responsibility should be to talk with him to attempt to determine what type person he is. Does he lack attention? Is he in need of a challenge? Is he depressed by the surroundings? What you tell him should not be based on how you feel, but rather how you would feel were you in his shoes, and what you could tell him to improve the situation. It could be a matter of telling him that geriatric care may seem unrewarding in many instances, but in actuality it is a very rewarding occupation, and why. It could be a matter of rephrasing a job responsibility in terms of a challenge, such as, "If you think that the work is really too much for you to handle . . ." Conversely, it may be a matter of stating, "You really are qualified for the work and don't let a couple of set-backs make you feel incapable . . ."

Obviously, the same rule can be applied to virtually any public or any person. The important thing to remember, however, is that just as an image must reflect a portion of yourself, and be accurate, so must the way in which you conduct interpersonal communications be sincere. For example, do not try to be a "back-slapper" if that is alien to your character, but do try to evoke those elements of your character which best befit both what you are trying to relate and the person to whom you are relating.

In some cases your ability in interpersonal communications will be called upon on the spur of the moment and you will be unable to methodically plan what you will say and how you will say it. But in those cases where a meeting is involved, or some other event for which you can plan, by all means take the time to determine:

> What type person you will be dealing with; what type information he seeks or what type motivation you will attempt to instill; and, what facts you will reveal and how you will go about revealing them.

What we are really talking about in terms of interpersonal communication is psychology, and this book can in no way go into the different types of personalities which exist and how best to relate to them. For this reason it is strongly suggested that some reading be done on the subject, or perhaps some courses be attended. The ability to empathize and then relate based on your understanding of your public's character is exceptionally valuable in every communications endeavor, and the expense of time on your part will be worthwhile.

VII

PHOTOGRAPHY

PHOTOGRAPHY IS A most important element of an overall public relations program which, unfortunately, few nursing homes utilize well. Photographs can be put to a variety of useful purposes; are relatively inexpensive, and can return benefits worth many times the expense involved, particularly in programs concerning employee relations, patient relations, patient family relations, community relations, and others. Consider the following brief list which illustrates how photographs can be used:

ACCOMPANYING NEWS RELEASES. A good photo with a news release increases the chance that your story will be used, if only through publication of your photo and caption.

FOR PATIENTS AND PATIENTS' FAMILIES. Photos of an event or activity are excellent for patient morale. A photograph of a birthday party placed on the bulletin board, for example, helps many patients remember the party and the pleasure it brought. Similarly, photos of patients can be sent to their respective families as proof positive of involvement and activity. Especially good photographs are saved and cherished, and the thoughtfulness of the sender is not forgotten.

FOR SCRAPBOOKS. Good photographs are essential for a scrapbook if it is to accurately portray activities undertaken in the nursing home. How many words would it take to accurately portray the enjoyment of fifty people at a party? Just one photograph shows it all at a glance, and probably much better than words could ever do.

FOR EMPLOYEES. Good photographs of employees, given to employees, are always appreciated.

FOR PUBLICATIONS. Photographs are excellent for "punching up" an in-house newsletter or for use with an article submitted to a magazine. In some cases the magazine may use the photographs, with credit, even if they don't use the article.

FOR DISPLAY. Good photographs of activities, framed, make excellent display material for office and lobby walls.

FOR TRAINING. In many cases photographs can be used for training new employees, illustrating the right way to perform a certain function.

FOR ADVERTISING. Photographs can be used in advertising as well as in brochures. Once again, they illustrate a point far more clearly and in far less space than words.

For Slide Shows. Photographs are easily converted to slides which can be used to make up a slide show on the nursing home, or as visual aids used in conjunction with a talk.

Establishing a Program

There are two general types of photographs you need if you are to establish a good stock photo library to draw upon whenever necessary. One type photo can be called "basic," illustrating specific facilities in use. The other type photo can be part of an ongoing program which chronicles special activities, such as parties, political rallies, special meals, and other events, as well as depicting various individuals involved. More explicitly:

Basic Photos. Basic photos include photographs of rooms and facilities in use, not just empty and dehumanized. Typical facilities include, where applicable: dining room; kitchen; occupational, physical and other therapy areas; lobby; grounds; several outside views of the nursing home, and so on. In cases where one area serves several purposes, such as a dining room which also is used as an occupational therapy area or movie theater, photographs should be taken for each use.

Ongoing Photos. Ongoing photographs should include photographs of special events such as birthday and holiday parties; barbeques, planting of spring flowers, outings, etc.; personal photos of certain patients doing things, as in occupational therapy, holding meetings, reading; photos of key staff members at work, including some relatively formal posed shots for use as author photos for magazines, or in announcing key staff promotions, etc.; photo of employees at work, and so on.

By establishing a program to take such photographs regularly, you should be able to create a stock photo library which covers the spectrum of your facility's activities and personalities which, in fact, comprise your nursing home environment. Above all, it is most important to carry on the program continually so photography becomes an integral element of your activities, and not merely an afterthought, sometimes forgotten when it should not be.

Assistance

In most cases it will be far too expensive to put a professional photographer on retainer to take all photos. It is strongly suggested, therefore, that you inquire of staff, patients and volunteers to determine who among them is a good amateur photographer.

While it would be ideal to have good photographs of all events, many ongoing photographs, especially those for use only in a scrapbook or on a bulletin board, need not be of professional quality. On the other hand, it is strongly suggested that a professional be hired to take most of the basic photographs and some of the ongoing ones. To locate a good photographer, utilize the Yellow Pages, ask friends or business acquaintances whom they utilize, or call a newspaper to speak with a photographer there. This latter method may be especially advisable if you wish to establish a connection at the newspaper. Bear in mind that newspaper photography often is not as introspective as the work of studio professionals and, therefore, newsphoto specialists should be led about to ensure that they capture on film exactly what you want to be seen. In many cases it is most economical to hire a photographer for five or six hours to shoot as many basic and ongoing type photographs as possible. Certain major events can be covered in a similar manner.

Equipment and Film

It is strongly suggested, in case of an in-house photographer, that a camera such as Kodak Instamatic *not* be used. There are several relatively inexpensive, almost foolproof 35-millimeter cameras on the market which can greatly enhance the quality and value of the photographs. Should the staff photographer not have such a camera, one could be purchased for the home.

You also may wish to obtain an "instant" camera, such as a Polaroid, in addition to the basic camera. The Polaroid concept of instant development is greatly enjoyed by patients. Do not rely on a Polaroid only, however. It is difficult and expensive to have duplicates made, and one of the prime purposes of photography is to establish a library reusable throughout the years.

Cost of film and developing, in the case of an in-house photographer, should be borne by the home. It is suggested that color film be used for other-than-Polaroid shots because, simply enough, you can make black and white prints from color, but you cannot make color prints from black and white negatives. When ordering prints, do not hesitate to ask for contact sheets only. In this way you can examine photos with a magnifying glass and determine which you want to have made into regular prints. There's no sense in paying for prints which will not be used.

As an adjunct to your photography program, consider incorporating photography into your home's activities program.

Taking Photos

Regardless of who is taking the photographs, several rules should be observed:

USE PEOPLE. Pictures of empty rooms or unused equipment are totally lifeless and give the image of dehumanization. A photograph of a room all prepared for a party, but devoid of people, is eerie compared to one in which the same room is shown bustling with activity.

TRY TO TAKE CANDID SHOTS. Candid shots usually are far more interesting than those in which the subjects are stiff and posed. In some cases it may be necessary to stage a candid shot, but even then it is possible to avoid the stiffness of a posed photo.

TAKE SEVERAL SHOTS OF AN IMPORTANT SCENE. If the scene being shot is particularly good, offering an opportunity for a one-of-a-kind photo, take as many shots as possible from different angles. In this way the chances for several superlative shots are increased, and a once-in-a-life-time opportunity will not be missed.

It is strongly advised that one of several available guides on photography, such as those put out by Kodak, be purchased. The cost is only a dollar or two; reading time is perhaps an hour at most, and the positive benefit in terms of improved picture quality can be immense.

Release

For legal purposes, it is essential that those photographed sign a photographic release or, in some cases, that a guardian or parent sign. A typical release form is shown in Figure 1.

For reference purposes, file releases themselves by number, and keep an alphabetical listing of signatures on 3 x 5 cards, each name followed by the number of the release. In addition, each photograph should be marked to indicate the numbers of the releases signed by those depicted.

Salvaging Photos

In some cases you may have on hand a photograph which is partly excellent, but partly bad. Bear in mind that the photo-

XYZ NURSING HOME PHOTOGRAPHIC PERMIT

I hereby authorize the taking of photographs of (name) and the reproduction and use of such photographs with or without identification, and without reservation by:

    A.   XYZ Nursing Home
    B.   The news media
    C.   Other (Specify): _____

    _____

Signature of responsible party or patient: _____

Signature of witness: _____

Date: _____

Figure 1: A typical photographic release.

graphic process is very flexible. Photographs can be cropped, or enlarged and cropped, to make them perfect for your purposes. For example, if an excellent photo of two persons is out of balance, the photograph can be enlarged slightly and cropped, so the two people appear in the center of the photo. Or if there is something undesirable in the background, the photo can be enlarged and cropped, or retouched. The retouching process—elimination of images in the photo by painting them out—can become expensive, however.

Creating a Photographic Library

Negatives of every usable photograph should be kept on file, each identified either by a negative number which you write on the wrapper, and/or by the edge number which appears next to the negative on the film. For reference purposes, so you can quickly determine what photos you have on hand and locate them quickly, keep a copy of each *print* in a notebook or box, printing on the back in grease pencil the edge number of the negative, and the numbers of appropriate photographic releases.

VIII

PRINT PUBLICITY

WHILE PUBLICITY IS an essential element of an overall public relations program, it should not be regarded as a be-all and end-all. It can serve a variety of purposes, not the least of which is letting your story be known to a general community, as through a local newspaper, or to more specific publics, through vehicles such as religious or trade publications.

An old PR axiom has it that "news is what an editor thinks is news." Do not believe that a story will be printed because someone knows someone at the newspaper. While such a contact helps, if a story is not newsworthy, it is useless. Of course, news is relative, and what one editor may deem worthy of page one will not even be considered by another.

The most common method for obtaining news media coverage is through issuance of a news release. While the most important element of a news release is the news it bears, certain mechanical considerations can be of utmost importance in the case of marginal releases, which most, in fact, are. As in so many other instances, it takes very little time or effort to do the job right, but few do.

Release Subjects

To expand on the "news is what the editor thinks is news" axiom, do not try to second-guess an editor by arbitrarily determining that a certain item is not newsworthy. Development and issuance of a news release is a relatively simple matter, and what you may have felt was not at all worthy of coverage might not only get published, but also may be used as a spark to the editor's own imagination, and lead to development of a story of large proportions. In other words, as far as issuing a news release is concerned, "when in doubt, do it anyway."

Typical release subjects are:

Changes of key staff personnel;
activities of staff members, including delivery of speeches, completion

25

of educational courses, promotions, publishing of an article, election
to officership of an association;

activities program happenings, primarily those involving all patients
(many of these releases could lead to excellent feature articles) ;

redecorating, new construction, and other changes to the physical
plant, and;

meetings to be held in the home, guest speakers, open houses, and
similar events.

In essence, all the above fall into the category of hard news, that
is, they are related to events and happenings. In fact, every event
and happening which occurs in your home, or related to employees, volunteers or patients, should be considered as the basis for a
potential news release. (In this regard, it also is wise to let employees and others know of your attitudes and encourage them to
submit information on events.)

Not all releases fall into the hard news category. As examples,
consider the opinion release which usually comes from the administrator of the nursing home, or other key personnel. It can be
based on virtually anything to do with health care, or with nursing homes or geriatric care in particular. For example, assume
that a bill pending before the United States Congress calls for national health insurance. Based on your own analysis of the bill,
or on others', you can write a release praising the bill, damning it,
offering changes, etc., simply by stating that you have "issued a
statement." Every quotation in the news release could then be
based on that "statement." Once the release is complete, write the
statement, which should be issued along with the release.

Similar to the above is the tie-in release based on material or a
release from a nursing home association, for example. Your release would cite your opinions coupled with those of the source,
with the source's statement or news release included along with
your own. In a similar manner, an item regarding national statistics or developments could be modified by you to take your own
community into consideration.

Still another type of release centers on statistics, involving development of figures regarding the number of patients who were
cared for during the last year; how much care was paid for by
Medicare or Medicaid (both nationally and in your own facility) ;
the total number of nursing hours put in last year by nursing

personnel, and so forth. Some of these aspects are discussed later in this chapter.

To go into all the possibilities regarding such events would take a full book, nor would it really be necessary. The best idea source of all are newspapers. Read as many as possible, and clip articles which you feel could serve as guides for your own releases.

Developing a News Media List

Essential to development of an effective news release system is compilation of a comprehensive news media list which includes pertinent information about each listed medium on individual 3 x 5 cards. In addition to the name and address of a medium, the following should be included:

DAILY NEWSPAPERS. At the very least, you should have a complete listing of all daily papers in your area including, for each, time of publication (AM or PM—AM papers are staffed most heavily in the evening, PM papers in the morning) and names of pertinent editors or reporters in health, geriatrics, science, etc.

WEEKLY NEWSPAPERS. The best way to establish a listing of local weekly papers is to consult your area Chamber of Commerce or state newspaper association. Various telephone Yellow Pages also will supply names and addresses. Listed information should include the day the weekly is published. (If a weekly is published on a Thursday, for example, releases for that edition should be in the editor's hands by Monday.)

PERIODICALS. Under the heading of periodicals, include all magazines produced within the state that concern themselves with health care, recreation and related matters, as well as local Sunday newspaper magazine sections. Information on each listing should include the date of publication and the name of pertinent editors.

RELATED PROFESSIONS' PUBLICATIONS. You should also include a listing of newsletters of all organizations to which you, other key staff members and your home belong as well as related organizations. Information should include the name of the person responsible for writing the publication and its date of issuance.

WIRE SERVICES. Include on your list the names and local office addresses of national wire services, including Associated Press, United Press International, and others. Frequently they'll be located at the offices of a major daily in your area.

MISCELLANEOUS PUBLICATIONS. You may also wish to include a list of miscellaneous publications which would be interested in certain activities of your home, key personnel or patients. This would mean, for example, church bulletins, alumni magazines, PTA newsletters, etc.

SELECTED WRITERS. Your list should also include certain free-lance writers whom you know to be active in the health care field. You probably will see their names mentioned frequently in various trade publications. Contact the publication's offices for the writer's addresses.

Your 3 x 5 cards can be filed alphabetically; alphabetically within media type categories (dailies, weeklies, etc.), or in any other manner which is convenient and most usable for you.

Writing the Release

While the writing rules advanced in Chapter V are generally applicable, press releases require a unique format and writing style, discussed immediately below:

FOLLOW BASIC STEPS. Basic to almost all forms of writing are the following steps: know your subject; assemble research material; read all research material at least twice; make reflective notes; categorize, all as discussed previously.

EVALUATE CATEGORIES. A press release must be organized on the basis of the most important subject first, second most important second, etc., much as a regular news article is written. This style is used because at times a story will simply be cut short by a newspaper's layout department, usually to make room for advertising. The cut is usually made as late in the story as possible, thereby leaving the most important elements of the article intact. For this reason, the subject matter of a news release should be evaluated on the basis of most important item first, second most important second, etc., with an outline developed in coordination with the evaluation.

WRITE THE LEAD. The lead, or first paragraph, is the most important part of the release. It should be a terse summary of the major elements of the story which lists the most important facts, usually in terms of answers to the questions who, what, why, when and where. To find examples of leads, pick up any daily newspaper and read the first paragraphs of hard news stories—not feature articles.

WRITE THE REST OF THE RELEASE. In writing the balance of the release, be certain to keep sentences as short as possible. Do not use any adjectives such as "wonderful," "terrific," and so on unless they are contained in quoted material. Such adjectives call for qualitative judgment, as compared to facts, hence must be attributed.

EXAMINE FIRST DRAFT. In examining your first draft, ask these questions of yourself: Have I said everything I want to say? Is all key information contained in the lead? Do subsequent paragraphs elaborate on the lead, most important item first? Rewrite and reorganize until each question can be answered with an unqualified "yes."

PREPARE FINAL DRAFT. In preparing your final draft, examine the release critically to ensure that sentences are as short as possible; that adjectives are limited and qualitative adjectives are in attributed quotes; that those quoted have given their permission to be quoted, and that all numbers, names and titles (including Miss and Mrs., college degrees, etc.) are absolutely correct.

Putting the Release on Paper

There is a very definite format you should use when typing up a release for submission. Examine the model release in Figure 2. The letters in parentheses on the release refer to the letters given below:

(A) STATIONERY. The release should be issued either on your home's letterhead or on special news release stationery which can have a large lettered "NEWS RELEASE" or "NEWS FROM . . ." printed across the top, centered, below being the name and address of the nursing home. In either case, it should be good quality paper. For best results, type the original on a blank piece of paper and duplicate onto your own stationery, *one side only*. This can be done with Xerox, Itek or similar equipment. If you do not have such equipment, contact a local printer. Only as a last resort should the original be typed on your stationery and then be duplicated together.

(B) TOP MARGIN. The top margin should begin approximately ⅓ of the way down from the top of the page, or at least 1½" below the letterhead.

(C) SIDE MARGINS. The left- and right-side margins should be 1½" from their respective edges throughout.

(D) CONTACT. "FOR MORE INFORMATION, CONTACT", should be the first line typed in all capital letters. Below that should appear the name, address and telephone number of at least one person who can answer quetions which a reporter or editor may have. You may wish to use two names, or include a home phone number for evening calls.

(E) RELEASE DATE. In most cases, the material you send can be published or reported at any time. In some instances, however, as in the case of an award to the employee of the year, you may wish to indicate that the release cannot be reported until after the event has transpired. This is most important for daily news media such as daily newspapers, radio and TV. In such cases, indicate the day on which the story can be reported, and the time—AM or PM. As an example, FOR RELEASE JUNE 17 AM. In the case of daily news media be sure the

(**A**) YOUR NURSING HOME'S LETTERHEAD
(**B**)
(**C**) <u>FOR MORE INFORMATION, CONTACT:</u>
John Doe
Doe Nursing Home
123 Main Street
City, State 12345　　(**D**)
Phone: 765-3421
<u>FOR IMMEDIATE RELEASE</u> (**E**)
<u>SMITHE NAMED EMPLOYEE OF THE YEAR</u> (**F**)

(**G**) <u>City, December 10</u>—Mrs. Jill <u>Smithe</u> (**N**),　(**H**)(**C**)
charge nurse of the Doe Nursing Home here
(**G**), has been named "Employee of the Year"
according to owner/administrator John Doe.

Mr. Doe commented that this was the first time
that presentation of the award was based on
balloting of all employees and patients. He said:
"We've been having the award for six (**I**) years
now, but we found a suggestion in the suggestion
box which gave us the idea to base the award on
what fellow employees had to say. Frankly, we
couldn't be happier."
(MORE) (**J**)
(ADD ONE) (**K**)　　　　　Doe Nursing Home/John Doe (**L**)
Mrs. Smithe stated that she was delighted that she
was selected. She said, "In the past some have
joked that the award was recognition of a 'teacher's
pet' and the winner was always in for a ribbing.
But this year, with the winner being chosen by 150
(**I**) people, employees, patients and volunteers,
it's a very, very gratifying feeling."
Mrs. Smithe is a registered nurse who graduated
from City High School and State College. She has
been employed by Doe Nursing Home since 1969.
(**M**)

Figure 2: Model press release

release is timed to arrive no more than three days before the release date.

(F) HEADLINE. A headline on a release is strictly optional, and serves only to alert the news media reader to the subject of the release. It's highly unlikely that a supplied headline will be used by the paper.

(G) DATELINE. If you do use a dateline, which seldom is necessary, it should indicate location and date of action, with action time references in the body of the release being based on the dateline time reference (today, yesterday, tomorrow) and location reference (here).

(H) SPACING. All copy should be double- or triple-spaced.

(I) NUMBERS. Spell out numbers one through ten, and use numerals for 11 and above. Never begin a sentence with a numeral.

(J) MORE THAN ONE PAGE. If the release is more than one page long, try to avoid ending any page in the middle of a paragraph, even if it means leaving an unusual amount of space at the bottom of the page. Be certain to include the word "MORE" in all caps and centered or to the right indicating that there is more copy. This should be done at the bottom of *every* page except the last.

(K) SECOND PAGE. On the upper left-hand corner of the second page should appear the words "ADD ONE", indicating it is the first additional page after the first. On the third page would appear "ADD TWO", and so on.

(L) RELEASE IDENTIFICATION AFTER PAGE ONE. At the top of each additional page, type in the name of your nursing home and the name of the contact.

(M) END SYMBOL. Indicate the end of the release by using, on the center of the page, the symbol # # #, or -30-, or -end-.

(N) PROOFREAD. Before the release is duplicated it should be proofread by at least two people. All numbers should be checked carefully, as well as spelling of names. In cases of long complicated names or unusual spellings of common names, underline to indicate to the editor that the name is spelled correctly, e.g., Papgoupolis or Smithe.

Mailing the Release

Attention should be given to who gets the release and how and when he gets it.

DETERMINE WHO SHOULD RECEIVE THE RELEASE. Go through your release list to determine what media should receive the release. Not all will be interested, but do bear in mind that releases can be rewritten so they will have great interest for certain media which otherwise would not care. You should differentiate by those media which *will* be interested; those which *may* be interested; those which *will* be interested *if* the release is changed; those which *may* be interested *if* the release is changed, and those which *will not* be interested under any circumstances. Do not mail releases to those media which will not be interested under any circumstances, and do not bother to rework the release if rewriting will net only a handful of maybes.

FOLD AND STUFF THE RELEASE WITH CARE. How you fold the release and stuff it into the envelope can be important, especially when dealing with editors and writers who are in a hurry, as most usually are. When folding the release, do it so the letterhead will be on top. In other words, place the release copy side down; fold the bottom edge to about 3⅔ inches from the top edge, then place the folded bottom on the top edge, and fold again. When stuffing into the envelope, the letterhead should be on the flap side, the first thing seen when the flap is opened. If a photograph accompanies your release, leave the release (and of course the photo) unfolded. Give extra support to the photo by including a piece of stiff cardboard with it and the release in a 9 x 12-inch envelope.

ADDRESS CAREFULLY. When addressing envelopes to media, be certain that each is desk- or person-directed. In other words, it should have on it either the name of a reporter or editor, or a title (e.g., Attn: Metro Editor) or both. This is especially important for daily papers. (See Chapter XVIII for information on mailing equipment.)

MAILING/DELIVERY. Once you have sealed your envelopes, determine when materials should be mailed by observing deadlines indicated on media list cards. If the release is particularly important, it may be wise to use a contact to deliver it in person, rather than sending it in "blind." Otherwise, be sure to allow enough time for the mailing process to ensure that the release will arrive no later than when it's supposed to.

Photographs

Whenever possible submit a photograph with your release. It heightens the chance of improved coverage, e.g., story plus photo plus caption versus story only, or captioned photo versus no coverage. It is imperative that the photograph be captioned for identification purposes. The caption need only be brief, serving mostly to identify what is depicted. A local newspaper should be studied for style. In cases where rather long captions are used with a story in a newspaper, but no general article accompanies the photo, chances are that only the photo has been used, and the caption is the only story to tell. In such cases the newspaper staff writes the caption, which is why yours must be utilitarian only.

Once you are certain that the caption is in complete accord

with the photo; that all names are spelled correctly, and that all titles, especially Miss, Mrs. or Ms., are correct, duplicate as many captions as there are photos. (Often you can type three captions to a page and in duplicating net three captions for three photos for every one page duplicated.)

Affix the caption to the photo by placing both face up; sliding the caption under the photo so the top of the sheet on which the caption is printed is approximately one-half inch above the bottom of the photo; taping the top of the caption sheet to the back of the photo, and folding the caption up so it serves to cover the photo. (See also Chapter VII.)

Tricks of the Trade

Here follow a few "tricks of the trade" which will improve your news release program.

MAKE THE RELEASE FIT THE MEDIA. Not all media will be interested in the same story, but be aware that many stories can be rewritten to fit the medium. For example, let's assume that employees select a patient of the year. The story going out to a daily paper will concentrate most on the person and the award itself. The same story rewritten for a newspaper from the person's home town would concentrate most on the recipient's past life in the local community.

EXTRA MILEAGE. Always be alert to the fact that extra mileage can be gained from a release concerned with one particular person by issuing the release to media concerned with the person involved, such as country club newsletter, church bulletin, alumni magazine, etc. This is not only a valued service which the person such as a new key staff member appreciates, but also one which will obtain even more mention of and knowledge of your nursing home.

QUOTATIONS. To emphasize a particular point, or to use adjectives which you would not ordinarily use in the body of a news release, create a quote. Make it interesting, and say it aloud to be sure it can be spoken without difficulty. Once you have the quote written, of course, contact the person quoted to ensure that you can use it.

EXCLUSIVES. If you see what you feel to be an excellent story developing, contact an editor and offer him an exclusive. Chances are he will send out a reporter to get the story, an investment he may have been unwilling to make if other news media also were covering the event. Make sure he does have an exclusive, but also be sure to issue releases on the same story once the first article appears.

SPECIALS. A special is not an exclusive. A special simply means that one particular version of a release is sent to one particular medium.

Be sure that such a release: is substantially different from any other on the same subject; is marked on the top "SPECIAL TO THE (Name of Medium) ", and is the original typewritten version of the release.

NOTES TO THE EDITOR. If an event is felt to be particularly newsworthy, attach a personal note to the editor with the release, the note going into greater, more informal detail as to why the material described is particularly important. You also may wish to extend an invitation to the editor or his representative to attend a certain function. Also, do not overlook the possibility of sending a note to an editor before an event transpires offering him an exclusive, or writing to give ideas about a possible feature story. For example, if you have as a patient a person who has led a very interesting life, or who was engaged in a now unused occupation, or who for some other reason is in your opinion worthy of coverage, send the editor a note with details of his past. You never know where it may lead to.

STATISTICS. Statistics are very cold and usually very uninteresting, but they can be made very interesting easily. For example, supposing your staff filled out 20,000 government forms in quadruplicate last year. This sounds like a reasonably large number but, rephrased, it could be "14 miles of government forms." Suddenly the flat statistic becomes much more active, alive and interesting through presenting it in a different light.

BEFORE AND AFTER RELEASES. To get extra mileage out of a good story, prepare a release which announces an event or program and when and where it will take place. Then, once it has occurred, send out a "wrap-up" release describing what happened.

ADDED MATERIALS. In certain cases, you will have available brochures and other material which, even though not pertinent to the release, can be included for the editor's use in whatever manner. If you are quoting from a prepared statement, enclose the full text to all media.

INTERVIEWS. In giving an interview to a reporter, keep several things in mind. First, know what you're talking about. If you're unsure of a name or statistic, don't mention anything until you can check it out. Second, do not preface any remark with, "Off the record." By doing this you annoy the reporter and, if he wants to, he may write in his article, "Mr. Smith told this reporter, off the record, that. . . ." If you do want something off the record, simply do not say it. Third, do not tell the reporter what to include in the article. If there are items you think should be covered, merely state that there are some other facts he may want to know about and indicate what some are. If he says he doesn't want them, so be it. If you force the issue he may interpret it as your telling him how to write, and you may be the loser because of it. (See also Chapter XXVI.)

PHOTOGRAPHS. Consider sending two or three photographs with a story instead of one, each, of course, being captioned. It increases the chances that at least one photo will be used, either along with or instead of a story. Also, if you have several acceptable shots and several local newspapers, consider sending each of two or three of the major papers a different photo, with still another different photo sent to all other area print media. With each of the one-of-a-kind photos include a note indicating that the photo is exclusive to the paper involved. Don't Bother a Writer or Editor. If you have sent a release to a paper or reporter, or if a reporter has been out to interview you, do not call to find out why the story has not been published. Such action will only irritate a writer or editor and diminish chances of publication. Buy Your Own. One of the greatest insults to a newspaperman is to ask him to send you clippings of an article, or a few extra copies when your story is published. If you want extra copies, buy them.

IX

BROADCAST PUBLICITY

BROADCAST PUBLICITY INVOLVES the same basic guidelines suggested for obtaining print publicity, in that news releases also should be sent to radio and television stations, which should be included in your news release mailing list. There are some basic differences, however, which should be observed.

Lists

You should have on file the names of radio and television stations which have their own news crews (in other words, a staff which does more than merely rewrite material as it comes off the AP of UPI wire) and their respective news assignment editors. Also determine and list which have locally-originated panel discussion or call-in talk shows and the respective program producers, personalities or talent coordinators.

Procedures/News

Just as you would give an exclusive to a newspaper, so may you consider giving an exclusive to a radio or television station. First, you must determine if the story really is worthwhile, because you will ruin your credibility (and wear out your welcome) if you call a television or radio station every time you have a release ready to issue. A worthwhile story, for example, would be a patient's 100th birthday party. To attempt to obtain coverage, call the news assignment editor of what you consider to be the best area television station. Introduce or reintroduce yourself and tell him that you think you have a story that would be of interest, and that you would be happy to give him the exclusive if he indicates interest. Inform him of the nature of the story and of the condition of the person involved. For example, if a patient is celebrating a 100th birthday, is in reasonably good health, alert, chipper, then chances are he will make for a good visual coverage. If interest is indicated, call no more stations and do not issue releases to any other television stations. Do prepare a release, however, as may be used for print media or radio, as well as a biographical summary sheet for use by the TV news crew. If no interest is indicated, try the next station.

The same procedure will work for radio stations, except the most important factor is how the patient sounds.

Of course, if you feel the story is "big," you may simply wish to send a release to all area TV and radio stations. If this tack is used, be certain to include a personal note to each news assignment editor indicating the condition of the patient(s) involved, possible angles, wry comments or particular opinions the patient may have, etc. Following issuance of the release by two days, call each editor to inquire if the release was received and, if so, if there is any interest. Expand on any comments made in the personal note, trying to excite the editor's imagination as much as possible. Do not go overboard. A news assignment editor is especially wary of overglamorized subjects or people, and you may very well run the risk of overdoing it and spoiling chances of success. Therefore, evidence your own enthusiasm but, as in all cases, stick to reality.

Procedures/Nonnews

Some of your best publicity may come from what is known as the nonnews category which, for the most part, hinges on your own ingenuity applied to radio and TV talk programs.

First assess each of the talk programs in your area to determine what type people and subjects they like to cover and what type audience is involved. It then will be up to you to come up with ideas, which you should send to the producer or talent coordinator in a personal letter. For example, you may be able to get together with other area administrators to determine if there are several patients who could appear on a talk show to discuss secrets of longevity, an always popular subject. You may wish to appear to discuss problems in selecting a nursing home. Watch for national issues as they may be applied locally. In some cases you may volunteer to appear on a program with someone who holds an opposite point of view. You may volunteer to appear with other health care professionals on the problems of aging and the aged, how best to care for these problems, and associated subjects. Read the newspapers and watch some of these programs for ideas. Whenever an idea does occur to you, write it down and follow it up with the letter. If you have no response in a week's time, call the person to whom you wrote. If there is no interest, keep trying.

You also may note that a particular reporter on a TV or radio station usually does a certain type story. If there is a way in which you can somehow develop a story in his line, call him up personally with your suggestion. Bear in mind that, for TV, visual impact often is as important as or even more important than the content. In this way a particular party being held in the home, with patients wearing bright, colorful handmade outfits and costumes may be excellent for TV while not at all that pertinent for radio or print media.

Also, be aware that both radio and television stations broadcast editorial comment. Particularly when the subject matter centers on problems with which you are familiar, immediately call the station requesting time for editorial response, providing you feel such response is in order.

A basic rule to follow in this and many other forms of PR is, if at first you don't succeed, try, try again. Eventually it will pay off. As a last word, don't forget national news and talk shows. If you have what you feel to be a particularly interesting story, do not hesitate to mail out a release or note. You never can tell what returns the investment of a postage stamp may bring.

X

LETTERS TO THE EDITOR

Letters to the editor can be an effective communications tool. For the most part, persons use them only when they wish to take a stand for or against an editorial, or to discuss what they feel to be erroneous reporting. But letters to the editor have far many more uses.

Some Typical Uses

Some typical uses of letters to the editor are as follows:

ANNOUNCEMENT. A letter-to-the-editor can be used to announce an event and encourage readers to participate in it, such as National Nursing Home Week, or an open house. (A press release usually is the preferred medium for such purposes, but the letter can be used instead of it if desired, or in addition to it.)

THANKS. A letter-to-the-editor can be used to thank a newspaper for coverage of an event, even if it only published the press release. Such a letter may not get published, but the editor will read it and appreciate it.

COMPLIMENT. Don't hesitate to compliment an editor or writer on an article in your field of expertise which you feel to have been very well done. For an example, an article on the plight of the aged which is well researched and written certainly merits your acclaim. The same applies to praise of an editorial.

CORRECTION. Send a letter to correct a misstatement or incorrect fact, whether or not it applied to you or your nursing home. In such a case remember that you draw more flies with honey than with vinegar. A strong statement blasting an editor for "this, that and the other thing" probably will never get published. A letter stated positively ("Mr. Jones did an excellent job of reporting, however, I believe there are several misinterpretations which bear correction . . .") gets much better response.

Do not overdo your use of letters-to-the-editor. If you do, your interest will be seen only as a desire to get your name in print. However, you should at all times write when the issues involved are germane, and when you have something reasonably appropriate to contribute or say.

Writing Your Letter

Writing a letter to the editor does not differ much from writing any other letter. Follow these simple guidelines:

OUTLINE. Be sure you create an outline which has an introduction, referencing the article or editorial, issue date, etc., with comments flowing in a smooth order, most important point discussed first.

WRITE. Write the letter based on the outline, keeping verbiage to a minimum. Hedge as little as possible. Be direct and forceful. Rely on the active tense, and keep sentences short.

EDIT. Try to keep the letter as tightly written and as brief as possible. If it requires too much editing on the part of the newspaper, it may be thrown out. Try to keep word count to no more than 500, usually two double-spaced, 8½ x 11 inch typewritten pages.

SUBMIT. Once written, submit your letter by mail. Clip the letter if published. In cases where you are announcing an event, the same letter can be sent to several publications.

Monitoring

An effective year-round campaign requires some monitoring of local media, reading the various local newspapers and magazines, and watching local news on television and listening to it on radio. Obviously, you cannot hear all the news, so be selective and, as far as broadcast media are concerned, try to watch only those which broadcast editorials. In most instances, both radio and TV stations with editorials will allow editorial response—a broadcast letter to the editor—from a responsible spokesman.

XI

BUSINESS LETTERS

Business letters often are very unremarkable forms of communication, except in cases where negative elements call attention to them and so create an unfavorable image. There are several excellent publications available on what should and should not be done, with the following points given to serve as reminders of key points to remember.

Outline

As with any other type of writing, first take notes on all items which you wish to mention in the letter, organize in terms of importance, and create an outline. In most cases just brief letters will be involved, and the outlining process, once established as a good habit, will be automatic.

Write

Working with the outline, write or dictate the letter, assuming the tone called for by the message conveyed. Keep sentences as short as possible, and try to make your point as quickly as possible, avoiding repetition. In cases of very important letters, have a draft written first and edit as necessary.

Proofread Carefully

In examining the letter before it is sent, proofread carefully. Putting your signature on the letter means you are responsible not only for what it says, but also the way it reads and looks. Check for misspellings, as well as for appearance, especially corrections. If there are more than one or two visible corrections, have the letter retyped. Also, if you note one or two mistakes in terms of what you have said or the way you have said it, don't be afraid to redo the letter. It is much better to take the time to create a more favorable impression. Do realize that if you are forced to do this frequently, however, you should do a better job in the first place, either by having a draft copy typed, or by editing the draft better.

Review Mechanical Procedures

It is good practice to occasionally review secretarial practices relating to letter writing. You should obtain and review any one of several available secretarial handbooks covering the subject. A typical business letter can be seen in Figure 3, with parenthetical letters referring to the items below. The format of the following sample letter is but one of several acceptable possibilities.

A The typewriter type should be clean and the ribbon should not at all be faded or worn. While slightly more expensive than a fabric ribbon, a carbon ribbon gives much better quality.

(B) The date can be placed in the upper right hand corner, three or four lines below the last line of the letterhead. In the case of a very short letter, the date, name and address should be placed lower on the page.

(C) Leave at least an inch or so margin on either side.

(D) The name and address of the addressee is placed on the left of the page approximately two spaces below the date, *not* using abbreviations for streets or states. In the case of letters going to a company, where a particular name is not known, you should add, after the address, "ATTENTION: Shipping Department," or whatever department is affected, beginning the letter with "Gentlemen:" or a similar salutation.

(E) The opening salutation should be formal, using the correct title, for those whom you do not know on a first name basis, or for letters of which copies will be sent. (A personal, handwritten note can be added to an original letter after copies are made.) In the case of a woman whose marital status is unknown, it usually is best to use a Ms. rather than a Mrs. or Miss, although the women's liberation movement, and some of the opposition it has engendered among the female ranks, renders this risky. If the letter is important, it is advised to perform minimal research to determine the correct title. Also, in cases of letters to congressmen and other governmental officials, you may wish to consult a dictionary which contains correct forms of address. In most cases, the opening salutation of a business letter should be followed by a colon (:) not a comma (,).

(F) If you choose to indent a salutation, indent all subsequent paragraphs. Likewise, a nonindented salutation, as illustrated, should be

(**B**) February 30, 1975

(**C**) Mr. John Doe
123 Main Street
(**D**) Anytown, Missouri 12345
Dear Mr. Doe: (**E**)

(**C**)

(**F**) In regard to your letter of February 24, 1975, (**G**)
I am happy to report that we do have
several beds available.

At this point in time, however, I am unable
to inform you whether or not our nursing home
is suited to provide the level of care required
by your mother as we do not have enough
specifics to make a judgment. There are a
variety of factors which must be considered,
both by us and by yourself. As a first step,
I would suggest that you consult with your
mother's physician or give us a call directly,
to determine the level of care required. If
skilled nursing care or intermediate care is
involved, we can be of assistance. But even
if the care we offer is the type required, I
strongly suggest that you visit our facility,
if possible with your mother, so we can discuss
all pertinent facts fully, and so you can see
what we offer and, generally, the type of care
we provide.

(**H**)
(**I**) Letter to John Doe, Continued

I am enclosing for your review a copy of our
brochure, a patient policy handbook, and
material on how to select a nursing home. You
may come in at any time, although I suggest
either making an appointment or calling ahead
if you wish to speak to me personally. On
occasion I am away from the home, but, of

course, competent assistants always are on
duty.
I look forward to hearing from you and to being
of service.

                    Sincerely,

                    William Miller, Administrator (**J**)

WM/abc   (**K**)

Enclosures (3)   (**L**)

Figure 3: Model business letter

followed by paragraphs separated by an extra space or two, nonindented.

(G) The opening sentence should reference the material about which
the letter is written, be it a letter, telephone call, personal visit, or
whatever. In some cases it is appropriate to add a line to the right of
and a line or two below the last line of the address, stating: REFER-
ENCE: Our order No. 12404, or whatever specific (other than a phone
call or visit or similar general matter) item is going to be discussed.

(H) If the letter will have to have a closing squeezed into the bottom,
or if just the closing, signature and related material is to appear on
the next page, it is better to retype the letter, beginning it lower on
the page, to permit at least three or four lines of copy to appear on the
next page, followed by closing materials.

(I) At the top of the second page, and on each succeeding page, should
appear wording identifying the letter, as illustrated, or similar.

(J) Include your title with your name. Usually it is best to include it
after your name, although others prefer it one line below. Also, some
prefer to include the name of the nursing home below the name and
title.

(K) The initials of the person dictating the letter should appear in
capital letters, followed by a slash line and the initials of the typist,
in lower case letters.

(L) If there are enclosures, the letter should so indicate, followed by
the number of enclosures in parentheses.

Carbon Copies

In case of carbon copies, be certain to include the full names
of those persons to whom carbons will be addressed. Also, you may
wish to mention in the body of the letter that carbons are being

sent, and, on occasion, you may wish to include a brief note with the carbon.

Blind Carbon Copies

A copy of a letter sent to a person not included in the carbon list on the original should be marked BCC, indicating that the letter's addressee does not know that a copy has been sent. A letter of explanation usually should accompany the blind carbon copy.

When Not Reviewing/Signing

In some cases you will dictate a letter which you will be unable to proofread or sign. In such cases your secretary should sign your name, putting her initials in parentheses. Also, you may wish to add, at the bottom and below typist's signature, DICTATED BUT NOT READ.

In all cases, you should attempt to get out a letter of response as soon as possible. Also, it may be wise to have your secretary keep track of those letters or other items to which you must reply and, if unanswered in a week's time, automatically type a letter stating that you are working on the situation and will reply shortly. All delayed responses should, of course, begin by apologizing for the delay. Also, consider using a short memorandum form, or even typing or writing a reply on the original letter itself, if called for, also stating something on the order of, "Please excuse the informality of the reply, but I felt you would appreciate the fastest possible reply."

XII

TELEPHONE TECHNIQUES

FEW ORGANIZATIONS OF any kind give telephone communication
the attention which it deserves. In essence, the person speaking
with a representative of your nursing home is deprived of four
of the five senses and must rely on his sense of hearing alone to
feed input to the imagination which, in turn, forms an image.
The scope and depth of the image depends on two variables: the
scope and depth of an individual's curiosity (more or less how
many blanks need filling in), and the strength of character (or
lack of it) evidenced by the voice from which the image is developed. The image developed can range from the very general (positive, negative or neutral) to the very specific (including the person's age, appearance, personality, etc.)

Perhaps most important, just as the voice is used to form the
image of a person, so is the image of a person used to form an
image of the nursing home he represents.

As an example, assume a call is being placed to a nursing home
with which the caller is unfamiliar. He is greeted cheerfully and
cordially and transferred to an individual who does his best to be
of assistance. At the very least, the caller's image of the home will
be positive, and he probably will have little hesitation about in-
vestigating establishment of a relationship with it. Conversely, if
the person answering the phone seemed devoid of emotion; if the
caller was transferred several times before finding an individual
capable of answering his questions, and if he was placed on hold
for several minutes and seemingly abandoned, chances are that
he not only would have hung up in disgust and not have called
back, but also that, given the opportunity, he would report nega-
tively on the entire organization, even though his appraisal was
based on the improper telephone technique of just two individuals.

If an organization is in the position of offering unique services,
it has little to worry about in terms of image. But, given the

46

amount of competition in the nursing home field, the amount of groundwork that is carried out by telephone, and the undeniable importance of first impressions, it becomes obvious that the necessity for correct telephone technique cannot be overemphasized.

Development of effective telephone technique is merely a matter of following a few simple guidelines, willingly adhered to once all personnel recognize that they are responsible not only for their own image, but also for that of the nursing home. Here follow the basic guidelines which, if observed, should ensure establishment of a positive image by telephone.

Receiving Calls

1. ANSWER PROMPTLY. The telephone should not be allowed to ring more than two or three times. Long delays in answering can result in an image of confusion, or of a generally unprofessional atmosphere.

2. LIFT RECEIVER STRAIGHT UP. When the phone is answered, the receiver should be grasped firmly and lifted straight up from the cradle to minimize chances of bumping it on the cradle or dropping it, either of which causes a loud, unpleasant noise on the other end of the line and creates an image of clumsiness.

3. AVOID CARRYOVER. Whoever answers the phone must avoid carryover of conversation or mood. Carryover of conversation refers to someone's finishing a conversation or comment while lifting the receiver, so the first thing the caller hears is something like: ". . . And have it taken care of today. Hello," which can be totally unsettling to someone relying solely on his sense of hearing. Carryover of mood is sometimes worse, and usually occurs when something has irritated a person immediately prior to his answering the phone, resulting in a terse, irritating, "Hello." In such cases, the person answering the phone should have the presence of mind either to compose himself before answering or have someone else answer.

4. RECEPTIONIST NEEDS CLEAR, PLEASANT VOICE. The duty of the person who is primarily responsible for answering a facility's phone (receptionist) is to make a caller feel welcome. Her voice should be clear and exude a cordial, competent, composed personality. Too often a receptionist will fall into switchboard syndrome where her voice sounds like that of a robot, and instantly conveys a feeling of cold impersonality.

5. RECEPTIONIST MUST GIVE OPENING SALUTATION. When the telephone is answered by a receptionist, an opening salutation such as "good morning" should be followed by the home's name stated fully and distinctly. If the home name is relatively short, it can be followed by, "May I help you?"

6. MODIFIED SALUTATION FOR NONCLERICAL. When the telephone is answered by someone whose job usually does not entail answering the phone, such as a nurse, the salutation should consist of the home name followed by the name of the person speaking, omitting the opening greetings. This is a simple method of letting the caller know that he is speaking with someone in a nonclerical position.

7. HANDLE TWO INCOMING CALLS CORRECTLY. If an incoming call conflicts with one already in progress, and if the receptionist cannot signal someone else to answer the incoming call, she should either transfer the first caller and then answer the incoming call, or ask the first caller's permission to be placed on hold ("Excuse me. The other line is ringing. May I place you on hold for a moment?") and answer the incoming call. The incoming call should be answered with the full salutation, not with, "Hold on please," or words to that effect. If the incoming call cannot be transferred immediately, and if the first caller still needs two or more minutes of attention, permission should be requested to call back the incoming caller immediately after the first caller is taken care of.

8. USE THE CALLER'S NAME. If the caller immediately identifies himself, as he should, his name should be written down and referred to during the course of conversation, if only to say, "Just a moment, Mr. Doe, and I'll connect you." This shows simple courtesy and efficient attention to detail.

9. DO NOT SCREEN CALLS. Calls should not be screened. When they are, the caller immediately realizes that someone is judging him, determining whether or not he is worth being spoken with. The potential time savings of such an approach clearly is not worth the potential harm which it may cause. It is advised, therefore, that honesty hold sway and the following rules be applied:

a) If the caller has identified himself, and if the requested party is known to be available, the caller should be told: "Just a moment, Mr. Doe. I'll get him for you."

b) If the caller has identified himself, but the requested party's availability is not certain, the caller should be told the situation: "Mr. Smith is in, Mr. Doe, but I don't know if he can come to the phone just now. I believe he's conducting an interview. Would you mind holding a moment while I check?"

If the requested party cannot come to the phone, the caller should be told: "Thank you for waiting, Mr. Doe. I'm sorry, but Mr. Smith is still tied up. Is it something that someone else could help you with, or would you like Mr. Smith to call you back? He'll probably be free in about a half-hour."

c) If the caller has not identified himself, and if the requested party is known to be available, the caller first should be informed of the requested party's availability and then be asked for identification: "Mr. Doe is in, sir. May I tell him who's calling please?"

(Note: "May I tell him who's calling, please?" is the most acceptable identification request. "May I ask who's calling?" can place a caller on the uneasy defensive (it's the standard line used in a screen) or, in some cases, it can anger a caller who feels that the secretary does not have to know who's calling. "May I tell him who's calling, please?" immediately identifies the reason for making the identification request and very gently reminds the caller that he should have identified himself in the first place.)

d) If the caller has not identified himself and if the requested party's availability is in question, the identification request should be made only after the caller has been informed if the requested party can come to the phone. If he cannot, but if another party can be of assistance, an identification request should be made prior to the transfer. If another party cannot be of assistance, and if the caller requests a return call, then his name and phone number should be requested. A caller should not be asked what firm he represents, although it is permissible to ask: "Mr. Doe, does this call refer to an ongoing situation so I can have the file in front of Mr. Smith when he returns the call?"

(Note: Some individuals attempt to screen calls by using a standard line such as, "Mr. Smith may have stepped away from his desk for a moment," prior to determining if the requested party wants to answer the call. While such a statement is permissible if true, bear in mind that any standard line is recognizable as a screen the second time it is used.

10. TRANSFER THE CALL CORRECTLY. When a call must be transferred from one office to another, the transfer process should be carried out in three steps:

a) The caller should be told why a transfer is necessary and his permission to make the transfer should be obtained: "Mr. Doe, I believe the best person to answer that question is Nancy Jones. Would you mind holding a few moments while I transfer you?"

b) The person to whom the call is transferred should be told who is on the line and why: "Mr. Doe is on line 28 about his mother."

c) When the person to whom the call has been transferred picks up the phone, he should greet the caller, identify himself, and apologize for the necessity of the transfer: "Hello, Mr. Doe. This is Nancy Jones. I hope you don't think we've been giving you the runaround."

11. DIFFERENTIATE BETWEEN CALLER AND SECRETARY. If a call is being placed by the secretary of a caller who will get on the line once the requested party is reached, the requested party should be told, "Mr.

Doe's secretary (or office) is on the line," not "Mr. Doe is on the line." Failure to make this differentiation could lead to embarrassment if the caller's secretary, and not the caller, is the recipient of a particularly hearty greeting.

12. 30-SECOND LIMIT FOR HOLD. If a caller must be placed on hold while a requested party is finishing another call, or while information is being gathered, or for whatever reason, his permission first must be asked ("Would you mind holding a few moments, please?") and he should not be left unattended for more than thirty seconds. At the end of that time, he should be informed of the status of his request, and status reports should continue at thirty-second intervals until two minutes have elapsed. At the end of two minutes, a call-back should be suggested.

13. KEEP THE CALL-BACK PROMISE. If a caller has been promised a call-back at a certain time, he absolutely must be called back at that time, if only to be told that the party or information he requested still is unavailable.

14. DON'T LEAVE TELEPHONE UNATTENDED. An unanswered phone can create a negative image of your home in terms of its ability to have sufficient personnel on hand. If there are occasions when your home's telephone may be left unattended during normal office hours, consider either an answering service or an answering device which utilizes a tape recording. In the latter case, a typical message is: "Smith Nursing Home. John Smith speaking. I'm sorry that there's no one in the office to answer your call right now. If you leave your message at the end of this recorded announcement, however, we'll do our best to have your call returned as soon as possible."

Placing Calls

15. DETERMINE WHO PLACES THE CALL. While most in the field seem to favor an individual placing his own calls, others argue, with reason, that it's a waste of time if the requested party is unavailable. The retort to that argument is that if the requested party is in, it is impolite to force him to wait while the caller comes onto the line. Perhaps an acceptable compromise for those who do not wish to place their own calls is having a secretary place the call with the caller picking up the receiver as soon as the requested party's availability is ascertained.

16. PREPARE BEFORE SPEAKING. Prior to placing a call, the caller should have before him:

   a) the name of the party being called

   b) the complete telephone number of the party being called (if the caller is placing the call directly)

   c) if necessary, an outline or checklist of points to be covered during the conversation

d) information pertinent to the call (files, etc.)

e) a reliable writing implement and paper

17. GIVE THE CORRECT OPENING SALUTATION. If the caller places the call directly, he should say, after the opening salutation on the other end, "Hello. This is John Smith calling from Smith Nursing Home. I'd like to speak with Tom Doe if he's in, please." (If the call is direct-dial long distance, the transferring process on the other end may be speeded if the caller adds the location of his firm, e.g., ". . . Smith Nursing Home in Omaha . . .")

If the call is being placed by a secretary, the opening salutation can be modified to: "Hello. I'm calling for Mr. John Smith of Smith Nursing Home (in Omaha). He'd like to speak with Mr. Tom Doe if he's in, please."

General

18. HAVE PEN AND PAPER BY EACH PHONE. A reliable writing instrument (such as a ballpoint pen), paper, and a telephone memorandum pad (which facilitates message taking) should be placed near each phone.

19. MINIMIZE BACKGROUND NOISE. Background noise such as loud music, voices, paper rustling, running water, etc., should be kept to a minimum. The telephone can pick up such sounds and make it almost impossible to hear on the other end, not to mention the harm which can be done to image.

20. SPEAK WITH NOTHING IN THE MOUTH. No one should speak on the telephone with anything in his mouth, such as a cigarette, cigar, pipe, gum or food. The telephone can amplify noises of smoking or mastication and create an unfavorable image of the speaker.

21. TALK INTO THE MOUTHPIECE. All persons should speak directly into the mouthpiece of the telephone receiver. Some persons have the bad habit of letting the receiver dangle so sounds are picked up more from the throat than the mouth. Such practice makes conversation difficult, while also creating an unfavorable image.

22. HOLD THE PHONE SECURELY. The receiver should be held securely while speaking to avoid the chance of dropping it. If you prefer to cradle the phone between ear and shoulder, a shoulder rest should be utilized.

23. SPEAK NORMALLY. Persons using the telephone should speak in a normal, conversational manner. Speaking too quickly results in a mumbling sound, while speaking too loudly can sound like shouting.

24. USE A COMPOSED VOICE AT ALL TIMES. It is essential that a business-like manner is reflected at all times through a composed voice which evidences cordiality and concern for the person on the other end of the line. If there is a situation which causes an obvious deviation from

this norm (such as anger, impatience, depression, etc.), the affected speaker should either apologize and offer an explanation, or ask to return the call at another time.

25. Avoid Artificiality. Artificiality is often conveyed by overcheerfulness or overconcern. The image projected is one of falseness, and hence can create distrust.

26. Use Hold Not Hand. At no time should a hand be placed over the mouthpiece of a phone. It indicates that someone is either shouting, saying something which he doesn't want the other party to hear, or just generally proceeding in an unbusinesslike manner. If a call must be interrupted to request information from a secretary, or for whatever reason, the caller should be given an explanation and placed on hold.

27. Double Check Information. All information should be double checked prior to closing a call. Spelling, in particular, must be gone over carefully, especially when it involves letters such as M's, N's, F's and S's, which are easily distorted by the telephone. The best method for verifying letters is to use common words beginning with the letters in question, such as "M as in mother," "N as in never," etc.

28. Hang Up Quietly. When a call is completed, the receiver should be cradled gently, or cradled only after the other party has hung up. A heavy hand easily is misinterpreted.

29. Avoid Immediate Comments. Some persons have the very bad habit of making comments about a caller as soon as the conversation is ended. On occasion, a person with this habit will make a comment prior to cradling the receiver completely, so the other party may overhear. If the other party happened to overhear a derogatory comment, the result can be disastrous.

XIII

SCRAPBOOK

A SCRAPBOOK IS AN excellent, low-cost public relations tool which can be used in a variety of ways. Consider keeping at least two types of scrapbooks, one to chronicle in-home activities, the other to record ways in which the home and its representatives relate to outside publics.

In-Home Activities Scrapbook

A scrapbook of in-home activities should contain photographs of noteworthy events, such as birthday parties, special evenings or dinners, meetings, talks, field trips, occupational therapy displays, and other events which are highlights of a year, as well as certain souvenirs such as holiday menus, issues of a newsletter or two, and related items. Such a scrapbook provides the prospective patient and his family with an idea of events in your nursing home, establishing a picture through photos and other items more effectively than words alone, and with far more substantiation. Also, such a scrapbook can be shown to virtually anyone interested in the home, including news media reporters, physicians, health inspectors, and others.

Outside Public Activities Scrapbook

A scrapbook for outside public activities should contain all the various news clippings about your home (including notes indicating TV and radio coverage), notices of talks (such as those appearing in the bulletin of a club or civic organization), photos of displays and personnel attending conferences, and related items indicating the home's and its personnel's involvement in the community in general, continuing education, and other activities and programs.

Type of Book

There are a variety of different type scrapbooks on the market. The one which seems easiest to use and most practical utilizes a plastic cover over a sticky page, enabling easy placement and re-placement of photos and other items and appropriate captions without glue and photo corners. A three ring binder to hold such material makes it easier to store and leaf through.

Keeping the Book Current

As with many other public relations programs, a scrapbook pro-gram is easy to undertake and maintain, providing someone does it. It is suggested that someone be assigned responsibility for each or both books, including taking photographs, and other "gather-ing" activities. People may look through your scrapbooks perhaps only a few times a year, but having a detailed chronicle available could be of inestimable importance.

The scrapbooks can be kept either on permanent display in the lobby, or in the office, and brought out to those waiting to see the administrator.

XIV

BROCHURE

Some nursing homes need a descriptive brochure more than others, depending on size of the home, vacancy rates, and related factors. Homes which have only an occasional need for a brochure often need little more than the copy, or writing, which would go into a brochure, neatly typed and duplicated onto nursing home stationery, used as an insert with a letter responding to an inquiry, for example. Given a relatively new home, or a large home, and a large amount of inquiries, however, a brochure will be far more effective.

While it is sometimes more expensive to utilize the services of a competent public relations firm to supervise writing, design and printing of a brochure, professional assistance is suggested strongly. Chances are that the finished product will be of as high a quality as possible within the working budget, and professional know-how often can result in cost-savings and/or quality improvement which the amateur would be unable to obtain. If retention of a PR firm is out of the question for the entire project, then at least consider use of professional assistance for certain portions of the work. Remember: A brochure is a salesman. Like all salesmen, it will be judged by how it looks and what it has to say. Unlike other salesmen, it cannot change the way it looks or what it says if experience determines a change is in order. Further, if the brochure is poorly done it presents a poor image, and the net result will be an expense of funds in an effort which actually is detrimental to the cause.

Preparing the Brochure

Following are many of the steps which a professional public relations firm would undertake in preparation of a brochure. If you decide to do it yourself, they also are steps which you must follow. Bear in mind that you can utilize professional assistance for at least part of the project, minimizing expense by relying on your own capabilities whenever possible. Also, be aware that you can obtain guidance simply by reviewing brochures of other nursing homes or, for that matter, of any type organization.

1. WRITE THE COPY. Following guidelines presented in Chapter V, organize the material you wish to include in the brochure. Information should be included about items which the public wants to know about, as well as those which you feel it should know about. A few typical sections might include:

a. *History of the nursing home,* including when it was established, the philosophy of management regarding care of patients, awards it may have won over the years, and other pertinent facts of general interest.

b. *Types of care offered,* including a listing and definition of levels of care, such as skilled care, intermediate care, and so forth. Be certain to include other names by which a level of care may be known, such as extended care, domiciliary care, and so on, to minimize confusion.

c. *Facilities,* including special rooms such as those for physical therapy, activities, reading; use of grounds; special X-ray or laboratory facilities, and so on.

d. *Staffing,* including types of nurses and their typical schedules, dietitians, volunteers, activities director, administrator, and other key individuals and personnel. *Do not mention anyone by name.* Doing so will quickly make the brochure obsolete if those named leave the nursing home.

e. *Accreditations,* including licensure of home, licensure of administrator, accreditations from government programs, membership in organizations such as the American Nursing Home Association or American Association of Homes for the Aging, etc.

f. *Miscellaneous,* including any special or noteworthy attributes of the home, such as facilities for preparing special diets, patient newsletter, or other items which are worthy of mention.

Naturally, the organization of the writing is up to you. You may wish to have only two or three general sections, or you may wish to break it down to a discussion of each department. Be careful not to include items such as costs and names which can change rapidly.

As a general rule of thumb, try to include everything you possibly can think of, realizing that it is a relatively easy job to delete material later.

Once the copy is in what you consider to be final form, have it read for comments by at least two people not affiliated with the home. Is there something omitted which should be discussed? Is there too much copy? Ask for a frank, critical appraisal.

2. DETERMINE A FORMAT. Once copy is complete you must determine

the format you want to use. The best method of doing this is to obtain as many other brochures as possible, not limiting yourself just to nursing home brochures. Three basic format sizes are 8½ x 11 inches; square (8" x 8" or 9" x 9"), or sized to fit into a regular business envelope, referred to as #10 size. The first two sizes (8½ x 11 inches or square) usually require covers and can be bound either with staples (saddle stitch), a plastic spiral binding, or a full plastic spine which slips over the cover and pages holding all together through pressure. The saddle stitch method usually looks and performs best. As far as the #10 size is concerned, it is easiest to mail and usually is a folded piece which, when fully expanded, requires only one piece of paper printed both sides, thus being the most economical to produce.

3. ESTABLISH A DESIGN. Assuming you have selected a format, the next step is overall design. Several designs should be prepared simply by sketching them on paper cut to the shape of the overall format. For example, if you have selected an eight-panel #10 size folder, meaning four three-inch panels to a side, use a 12 by 8½ inch piece of paper, the 12-inch edge being horizontal and folded twice to achieve 3 by 8½ inch #10 size. Photographs or other illustrations, including one of the home and another of patients and staff, should be indicated, as well as each section "head," that bold type line which indicates what will be discussed in the copy immediately below.

4. SELECT COLORS. Obviously, a full-color brochure is an elegant publication, but one which is comparatively expensive. On the other end of the spectrum, expense can be minimized through use of only one color, but the product sometimes suffers as a result. Nonetheless, professionals are able to design one-color brochures which not only are very attractive, but which also give the impression that several colors are involved. Here are some of the professional tricks of which you should be aware.

a. *Colored stock,* meaning colored paper, comes in just about every color imaginable. Usually colored stock looks much better than plain white paper, and in some cases costs less.

b. *Reverse printing,* which means that the actual printing comes out the color of the paper, the ink being used to go around the letters. In essence, it is like using the negative of a black and white photograph.

c. *Screens,* meaning using the ink at less than full intensity. For example, black ink screened at 50 percent results in gray. Ink can be used at full strength and at screened intensities on the same brochure at no additional cost.

d. Color combinations can result when two colors are used. All for the cost of two inks only you can achieve the color of one ink; the color of the other ink; the color of each when screened; the colors which result when the two inks are mixed together at full strength and at different intensities. Even more coloration can be achieved when colored stock is used.

Always bear in mind when selecting colors that photographs will be shown in the ink colors selected. In some cases, therefore, it may be best to use sketches or line drawings instead of photographs. A sketch can be made quickly and easily by placing tracing paper over the photograph. Inexpensive professional assistance can be obtained from a teacher at a high school art department, or from an artist at a local daily newspaper art department. Likewise, type must be easy to read. If you choose only one color, be sure it will result in easy reading.

5. SELECT PAPER. Assuming you know what colors you are interested in, the next step is to select the paper. A sample of papers may be seen by calling a paper house (under "Paper Products" in the Yellow Pages) which probably will be happy to send you several different swatch books. Paper samples also can be obtained from a printer, if you already have one in mind. Your selection of paper should be based on quality and colors available. If you want only a small quantity of brochures you would be well-advised to select the best paper available as high quality stock costs little more in small quantity. On the other hand, if many brochures are required and the budget is limited, a lower grade of paper may be advisable.

6. HAVE DUMMIES PREPARED. Once you select the paper (or papers if the brochure is to have text and separate cover), call the paper house or printer and request several dummies which will be cut and prepared to the dimensions you want, utilizing the paper you have selected. Sketch in your intended design on one of the dummies.

7. SELECT A PRINTER. The next step is to select a printer. Write down all your specifications, including the number of half-tones (photographs), size and type paper, and the quantity. Tell the printer that copy will be camera-ready, even though at this point it is not. A good printer should be able to get back to you in a day, and some will be able to give you a price while you wait. Do not necessarily select the low bidder. Rather, choose that one who you feel will offer the most value for your money, who can deliver quickly and who can assign someone to work with you.

8. SELECT TYPE. Once you have selected a printer, visit with him to determine what type styles he has in-house. In most cases supply will be limited. If you can find a style for text copy and heads, fine. Otherwise, ask to see type catalogues available from various type houses. The printer should have them on hand. In selecting type, bear in mind that the style selected for the head has much to do with the overall appearance of the brochure. It can be very modern, if this is the image you wish to convey, early American, traditional, or what have you.

On the other hand, the body type should be selected on the basis of legibility. Consider making the type you select larger than usual to permit easy reading. It's much wiser to cut your copy or change format than to produce a relatively illegible brochure which will go unread.

9. FINAL PREPARATIONS. Before proceeding to the finality of printing, several steps must be taken:

a. *General evaluation* should be performed by the printer. Allow him to make suggestions regarding all phases of your brochure, including design, color, paper and so forth. Also, be sure a word count is taken to ensure that your copy fits the format. If not, either change the format or cut the copy.

b. *Mark-up copy for type,* which means indicating what size type to use, what margins are involved, what spacing there should be between lines, and so forth. This job is best done by a professional. While you feasibly could leave it to a free-lancer or moonlighter (if one was involved at the design stage), it is least confusing when handled by the person responsible for setting type. Whoever sets the type also could be responsible for laying it out on the page, ready for printing.

c. *Last reading* should be performed prior to the copy's being marked-up for type. This must be a close reading because changes made after this point are costly. Be sure everything is said exactly the way you want it said; that all spellings are correct, and that any and all corrections are indicated clearly.

d. *Proofread the galleys,* or pages of type as they come from the typesetter before being laid out. This will help ensure that any typographical errors are caught before they are pasted up.

e. *Check the paste-up,* that stage of production in which the type is pasted into position prior to being photographed for the making of photo offset plates. Examine either the original paste-up ("boards"), or a copy of it.

f. *Check the proof,* in photo-offset usually referred to as the "blue line," looking for scratches on the photographic plate, dust specks, etc. At this point there should be no need for making any changes to the text or layout.

Once the Brochure Is Complete

Once you have the brochure, it is your responsibility to ensure that it remains current. If major events transpire which cause the brochure to be inaccurate, another should be prepared, often by making textual changes which easily can be accommodated within the current design of the brochure. In some cases, rather than reprinting, you can have a gummed label made up which can be neatly placed over obsolete copy, thereby giving you the effect of a new brochure at a very minor cost.

When mailing the brochure, never send it alone. Always accompany it with a personal letter which answers any specific questions which a person may have asked, such as rates, and so forth. At the very least, thank the person for his interest and invite further inquiry.

XV

PATIENT POLICY HANDBOOK

IT IS ESSENTIAL to have a patient policy handbook which sets forth rules and regulations concerning your nursing home. The primary publics for such a handbook are patients and their families, with secondary publics being employees and volunteers, as well as prospective patient families.

Contents

Contents should cover as many elements as need to be covered, such as those which follow:

INTRODUCTION. The introduction to the piece, which should appear on a separate page, sets the tone for the rest of the book. It should emphasize that rules have been established primarily to further patient care and provide for patient safety and well-being. You may wish to consider one standard introduction aimed primarily for patients, with an additional insert for patient families. Typical patient-directed copy is as follows:

This handbook has been prepared to provide you with information on Doe Nursing Home and the rules and regulations we have established to help ensure your fellow patients' well-being. If you have any questions or comments at any time, please feel free to tell us. It is our purpose to serve you, and help whenever we possibly can.

Typical copy, for reading by patients' families, is as follows:

This handbook has been prepared to provide you with information concerning patient care policies of the Doe Nursing Home.

Administration and staff of Doe Nursing Home make every effort to ensure the comfort and well-being of those entrusted to our care. Through a variety of programs, we endeavor to help each patient achieve as great as degree of independence and self-reliance as possible. While complete rehabilitation seldom is possible, it is a goal toward which we continually strive. It is our proudest accomplishment when a patient can leave our care and return to the community, able to cope with the many requirements of daily living.

One of the prime requirements in a program of patient care is the patient's own desire to get well. This requires a healthy emotional outlook, something you can help with through frequent visits, let-

61

ters and calls. A patient easily can interpret confinement in a long-term care facility as abandonment by loved ones, so continued interest in patient care and well-being is essential.

It is very important to bear in mind that a patient is an adult individual. At times statements will be made which are intended to make family members feel guilty, or which are intended to elicit sympathy. For example, new patients often will make complaints about lack of care and attention which are contrary to fact. We do not mean to discount such complaints. In fact, we request that any complaint immediately be brought to our attention. But do realize that in some cases complaints center on problems which do not exist, while serving to point out an emotional problem which may exist. As an example, continued complaints of lack of care, when care is comprehensive and thorough, may be the patient's way of urging you to visit more.

Please read this handbook thoroughly. If you have any questions, please feel free to contact us at any time.

VISITING. This section should encourage visiting as frequently as possible, and also should indicate when visiting hours are; visiting hours in rooms as compared to lobby, etc.

GIFTS. This section should indicate the value of a patient's receiving an occasional gift; what type gifts may most be appreciated and who in the home a family member could contact for advice in selecting a gift; what type gifts should be avoided (such as tobacco, certain foods, etc.) and related information.

FIRE SAFETY. A section on fire safety should indicate precautions taken by the home to prevent fire and deal with it should it occur, as well as precautions which visitors should observe, such as not smoking in patients' rooms, and so forth.

TIPPING. The nursing home should establish hard-and-fast policy regarding tipping, preferably against.

EXTRA SERVICES. This section should specify the most commonly used extras, such as special duty nurses, physical therapists, special diets, wheelchairs, etc., advising further that virtually any special requirement can be met.

PHYSICIANS. Clearly detailed information should be given on arrangements with physicians; whether or not a patient's personal physician can be used, etc.

MEALS. Explaining how many meals are served per day and when, meal planning and who does it, etc.

EXTRA COST ITEMS. Including activities programs materials, canes, wheelchairs, and so on.

EMERGENCY MEDICAL CARE. Detailing with what hospitals the nursing home has transfer agreements, usual emergency procedures, etc.

PAYMENT FOR CARE. Touch on the home's willingness to assist in determining eligibility for assistance from federal or state programs; when payment is due, what happens if payment is not received, and related information.

COMPLAINTS. Request that they be brought to the attention of an appropriate party.

Additional information can be included as experience indicates. Other information, to an extent answering questions which may be asked, can be included based on material discussed in the various selection guides intended for consumer use.

Appearance

The most important element of the handbook is what it says, not necessarily how it looks. Some general considerations regarding appearance, however, are these:

1. *Use large type,* to ensure easy reading by patients. In the case of a typewriter, use either the IBM Orator font or all capital letters.

2. *Make it neat,* when using typed pages by placing it into an inexpensive but relatively attractive binder. If printed, consult your printer for a workmanlike, but not elaborate design. Chances are that there will be frequent revisions so expending a great deal of money for design and other elements could become very costly.

3. *Have it printed in quantity,* so it can be distributed freely to patients, employees, volunteers, patient families, and to those who are seriously considering use of your facility. Never give out a used copy.

XVI

BULLETINS

A T TIMES THERE will be a need to disseminate news to employees, or patients, or others in the nursing home in a hurry, or at a time when other methods (such as the newsletter or bulletin board) will not be responsive enough either in terms of time or audience reached. For this reason you should consider establishment of a bulletin form which allows you, or a department head, or others to create a notice that is quickly identified and easily distributed.

A typical bulletin form, printed on inexpensive white paper, would have the word BULLETIN (or Actiongram, or whatever) printed in large, bold letters across the top, TO:, FROM:, and RE: printed one above the other below the headlined word and about an inch-and-one-half from the left margin, and DATE: printed on the same line as TO:, but about three inches from the right margin. All printing can be done in bright red to make the piece highly visible. This standard form makes it easier for general purpose in-house communication when it must be done in a hurry.

Use of the Bulletin should be available to all appropriate personnel, with the "FROM:" being responsible for disseminating it to the "TO:". All able to use the bulletin should be reminded not to abuse it by using it for less than urgent or fast-breaking news. Otherwise it will lose importance and will be disregarded by those who should be reading it. In other words, don't "cry wolf."

XVII

NEWSLETTER

RELATIVELY FEW OF the nation's nursing homes have undertaken establishment of an in-house newsletter. One probable cause for not using this excellent PR tool is apprehension that the tasks involved are too many and too complicated, and/or that the costs are too high. The facts are, however, that establishment and regular issuance of an in-house newsletter can be a very uncomplicated, inexpensive project whose benefits far outstrip the effort involved.

The in-house newsletter serves two basic purposes. First, and most obviously, it is a communications device which informs readers of what is happening in the nursing home. Second, and perhaps more important, the newsletter treats the nursing home as a whole, and in familiar, informal terms, thereby unifying its many elements while creating a sense of family and realization that the nursing home, after all, is a community of people, and not merely an assemblage of bricks, mortar, and nameless faces.

It is not especially important that your newsletter look like an expensive, professionally produced publication, nor that it be written as if the editor were trying for a Pulitzer Prize. In fact, if the establishment of intimacy is a goal of publication, as it should be, an overly "slick" appearance can be detrimental, possibly appearing as aloof, cold and uninvolved.

There are several types of newsletters which can be considered, including: a general newsletter covering all aspects of home activity; a patients-only newsletter; an employees-only newsletter, and a volunteers-only newsletter. Some homes, if large enough, feasibly could have one of each, the general newsletter being primarily for those not actually in the home. In most cases, however, it is strongly recommended that the general newsletter type be selected with, if necessary, an insert sheet of job-related news exclusively for employees, with possibly another for volunteers. For the most part, it is the general type newsletter which is discussed below.

Setting a Budget

The first step toward establishing a newsletter is the setting of a budget, and in so doing establishment of other basic criteria.

It is suggested that allocating a small, minimal budget at the outset will be effective. It will allow you and others involved to gain valuable trial-and-error experience at small cost, while also permitting steady improvements in the newsletter's appearance. With this in mind, consider that your basic format should be typed only and without photographs, with the newsletter being published on a monthly basis.

The basic costs involved in such an approach will be:

1. EDITING. If you choose to utilize outside talent it should cost no more than $20 or so per issue. In most cases, outside editorial talent is not essential.

2. TYPING. In this case, typing automatically includes layout, which can be undertaken in house by a secretary.

3. PRINTING. If you have in-house equipment, such as a mimeograph or Xerox machine, determine how much in-house printing will cost before assuming that it will be the least expensive method. A local printer may be able to do the job for substantially less. Naturally, if patients would be involved in use of in-house equipment, the involvement and feeling of accomplishment they achieve also must be considered. Factors to include for determination of printing cost include amount of pages and amount of newsletters to be printed. You should allow some five pages per issue, with number of copies to be printed based on those you intend to distribute the publication to, such as:

    patients;
    employees;
    volunteers;
    patient families;
    former patients;
    former patients' families;
    government officials;
    local, state and federal legislators;
    members of the community health care public;
    related associations, and;
    other nursing homes.

4. ASSEMBLING. Collating the pages and stapling them together can be done by the printer for a fee (assuming he does the actual printing), or it can be a task assigned to patients.

5. ADDRESSING. Envelopes for those to whom the newsletter is to be

mailed can be addressed by hand by patients or staff. If more than 25 newsletters are being mailed per issue, however, it is recommended that addressing equipment be utilized, as discussed in Chapter XVIII. If addressing equipment is used, determine which costs or portions of cost, as for equipment, supplies and possibly address plates, will be allocatable directly to the newsletter. Bear in mind that the bulk of initial expense for mailing equipment will be one-time only, with much of it assignable to other projects for which it also will be used.

6. INSERTION. Folding and stuffing of newsletters into pre-addressed envelopes can be performed by the printer or by patients or staff.

7. POSTAGE. Mailed newsletters should be sent first class although, if the budget is tight, third class bulk is acceptable. (Nonprofit homes may be able to utilize a special nonprofit bulk mailing rate.)

Assuming a distribution of 250 five-page newsletters 12 times per year, with 100 mailed first class each issue, there is no reason why total annual costs cannot be kept below $350, or less than $30 per issue, a very small price to pay for a program which has many positive effects on many different publics.

Initial Meeting

Once basic budget and related data are gathered, it is advised that an initial meeting be held with representatives of employees, patients and volunteers. They should be informed that the home will be undertaking regular publication of a newsletter; that it will be an effective communications tool for all parties concerned, and that it should generate involvement and enthusiasm. At this time certain elements discussed below can be covered, or you may wish simply to distribute material for study prior to a subsequent meeting, giving representatives time to think about the subject and discuss it with others.

Organizational Framework

It is imperative to establish some sort of organizational framework for newsletter production to determine who shall be responsible for what. Several alternatives should be considered. The newsletter can be the responsibility of someone on staff or a volunteer, or can be assigned to someone hired (on a free-lance basis, for example), who would gather news stories from various sources and then write the entire publication. This method obviously limits involvement. A second method involves dividing the newsletter

into distinct areas of responsibility, with an employee responsible
for gathering employee news; a patient responsible for gathering
patient news; a volunteer responsible for volunteer news; a management representative responsible for gathering job-related news
for a separate insert, and the volunteer director responsible for a
volunteer-only insert. This is an excellent method, in terms of
involvement, providing that "responsibilities" are not taken to
mean doing everything on one's own, but rather delegating as-
signments, so that within each news public category a variety of
tasks are assigned to all willing to participate, particularly on the
patient side (which involves participation with an activities program). A third method would make the entire production an element of the patient activities program, with patients responsible
for all tasks with the possible exception of typing and printing.

In establishing either of the latter two methodologies, it would
not at all be inappropriate to call on an editor of a local newspaper, daily or weekly, to visit the nursing home particularly to
help patients organize and develop the program.

For the purposes of this chapter, we shall discuss the second
type approach, which has implications for both the other methods.

Possible Topics

It is of course important to determine what type articles will be
included in your newsletter. Here follows a descriptive listing of
some of the most popular possibilities.

> EDITORIAL. An editorial, from the administrator, department head, or
> patient, may take the form of a regular column, each issue beginning
> with FROM THE ADMINISTRATOR, or it may be a changing
> column, one month featuring an editorial by the administrator, the
> next from a patient, the next from the dietitian or activities director,
> and so on. You also should consider going outside the home seeking
> an editorial from your congressman or mayor. The subject matter for
> an editorial can be wide-ranging, from concepts of aging and the role
> of the nursing home to international relations.
>
> LETTERS TO THE EDITOR. This is an excellent newsletter section to con-
> sider, especially if you run editorial matter.
>
> PRO AND CON. Similar to an editorial, this feature involves two people
> each writing positively about his own position on a certain given
> issue, the two viewpoints being diametrically opposed. The important
> point to remember for this type article is that each writer must write

positively about his viewpoint, and must *not* be derogatory toward the "opposition's" views.

HUMOR COLUMN. Humor is a wonderful gift which should be shared. In-house humor perhaps could be written by a patient. A column title, something like "What Annie Heard," could comprise humorous and harmless anecdotes and gossip about patients, employees, and volunteers, or about the world in general. Bear in mind that such a column calls for a writer able to write in the style required.

NEW PATIENTS/EMPLOYEES/VOLUNTEERS. Such columns provide brief biographical material not dissimilar from small articles seen in daily newspapers.

EMPLOYEE/PATIENT/VOLUNTEER OF THE MONTH. This can be a regular spotlight feature providing in-depth biographical data, information on hobbies, interest, growing up, opinions, etc. of the Employee-, Patient- and Volunteer-of-the-Month. As discussed in Chapter XXXI, the persons featured in such spotlight articles probably are best chosen on a random basis.

CURRENT AND COMING EVENTS. Articles on what's happening comprise the hard news element of the newsletter, through articles telling about upcoming programs, special meals, parties, events, exhibits, displays, trips, and so forth. The extent of detail given to each item depends on its relative importance, and the length to which you wish to keep the newsletter.

DEPARTMENT NEWS. Providing news department-by-department is similar to the above, merely presenting what's happening in a more compartmentalized manner.

PERSONALS. Columns relating personal information should treat all personnel as a group rather than breaking the section down by employees, patients or volunteers. Brief run-on information on birthdays, anniversaries, weddings, bereavements, news of former patients or employees, and so forth should be provided. There should be some limit on this type column, however, as it can develop into one of the major elements of a newsletter, which it most definitely should *not* be.

MISCELLANEOUS. Whenever possible, the newsletter should contain filler material such as poetry, jokes, cartoons and similar items.

CLASSIFIED ADVERTISING. A classified advertising section is suggested for use by employees and volunteers, either as a separate insert or as part of an employee-only and/or volunteer-only insert, allowing employees and volunteers to advertise, at no cost, items sought or for sale.

Inserts

An employee-only insert, mentioned above, is primarily the responsibility of management. It can contain directives, changes of policy, and related material of interest strictly to employees.

One caution should be observed. When putting down policy directives in black and white, there is the inevitable tendency for them to appear very strict and cut and dried. For this reason, it is advised that they be softened to as great a degree as possible, without, of course, weakening the message. For example, rather than saying, "All employees must be on time to assume their shift duties or else will be docked in pay. Repeated offenses will result in dismissal," consider the same message gotten across as follows:

> "We have noticed of late that some employees are coming in late for their shifts. This creates the risk of endangering the quality of patient care we have become known for. It can leave us understaffed, on occasion seriously so. Chances are we will not have an emergency situation arise right after we change shifts, but what if we did? The great responsibility we have for caring for those who hardly are able to care for themselves fully demands that we do our best to fulfill assigned duties. Also, those who come in late are being unfair to fellow employees; to those who are conscientious enough to stay on those extra minutes, and to those who make every effort to be on time. To encourage on-time reporting, we have decided, in conjunction with the Employees' Council, to have late arrival reflected in paychecks and, if necessary, to take stronger action, including discharge. This should not be taken as a threat. Rather, it is a plea that you recognize your responsibilities of caring for those who are relying on you for care and protection."

In essence, the same thing has been said, but it now is accompanied by an explanation, and is written in such a manner as to encourage employees to be on time because they *want* to be on time, not just because they may lose pay or get fired if they don't.

The employees-only section also could include an administrator's message, perhaps a continuing feature pertaining primarily to patient care and employee attitudes toward patients. An Employees Council head also could have a column.

A special insert also can be made for volunteers, by the director of volunteers or volunteers and activities, which could discuss certain management issues only, rather than those bits of news which are germane to general readership, such as upcoming programs, award of hourly pins, and so forth.

Assigning Responsibilities

It is to be expected that management methods utilized to gather news will vary markedly from home to home, each being subject to trial and error; each finally evolving into an effective method given the personnel within a given home. Therefore, the following guidelines should serve as a model only, to be modified as situations and experience dictates.

As a possibility, it is suggested that three employees (unless more can be found) be generally responsible for gathering employee news, and possibly editing it. Each of the three should have one or two department heads assigned to him and, in turn, department heads should be responsible for at least writing notes relating to personal news within the department as well as current or planned events. In this way department heads can be contacted before the deadline approaches, to expand on the notes submitted. Likewise, several patients, and possibly some volunteers, should be assigned duties of getting news stories regarding patients, dividing reportorial duties by rooms or areas.

In a similar manner, a volunteer or two could be responsible for gathering news regarding volunteers.

As an adjunct to news reporting, certain persons may be appointed specific responsibilities, such as writing the employee/patient/volunteer-of-the-month spotlight features, or new patients/employees/volunteers biographies.

It probably is advisable also to have an overall editor-in-chief, responsible to the administrator, who would review all materials and edit as required. This person probably can be found among the ranks of persons in the home, and would be mostly responsible for grammar and brief items. In addition, the editor-in-chief would act as the overall manager-coordinator, responsible for assuring that the various elements are gotten together on time. An overall editorial board, carrying representatives of administrators, employees, patients and volunteers could meet monthly or quarterly to determine new features, who should be solicited for guest articles, and other material.

As can be seen, use of this model encourages participation throughout the home which, we believe, is a positive goal.

Space

To help assure smooth production, some space must be set aside, if only shared space available only at certain times. In cases of newsletters produced primarily or exclusively by patients, a small room may be given over exclusively to the newsletter to help give a "something special" quality. At the very least, there must be one central location at which all the various stories, ideas for stories, etc., can be kept, if only space in an office file drawer.

Setting Deadlines

The setting of a deadline is a "working backwards" affair which establishes a coherent timetable in its wake. For example, if the newsletter is to be issued on the last day of the month, the following timetable could evolve:

DAY NO. 30, AM—Issue Newsletter
DAY NO. 29, PM—Collate, fold, staple and stuff
DAY NO. 29, AM—Address envelopes, receive newsletter from printer
DAY NO. 28,—Print
DAY NO. 27, PM—Review and correct proof sheet
DAY NO. 27, AM—Type up newsletter
DAY NO. 26, PM—Type up newsletter
DAY NO. 25, PM—Proofread submission to typist
DAY NO. 25, AM—Editing
DAY NO. 24—Gathering last minute stories and editing
DAY NO. 23—Gathering last minute stories and editing
DAY NO. 22—Editing

The above, of course, is a simulation only, and one which does not take weekends into account. The schedule you establish will have to be based on the time it actually takes to perform certain functions. But as the simulation does show, by working backwards you will be able to establish a time-table enabling those involved to know what has to be done and when it must be done.

Type and Layout

It is suggested that, at least at the outset, the newsletter be typed, rather than set in type. This is the least expensive method and proves highly readable. If an IBM Selectric typewriter is available, it is strongly suggested that the special Orator font be obtained. It utilizes extra large characters which are easily read by patients. If such a typewriter is not available you should consider typing with all capital letters.

The simplest form of layout, given an 8½ x 11 inch sheet, which is recommended, involves: leaving at least a one-inch margin on either side; typing the headline and complete story, then leaving four or so spaces between stories. Recommended headlining procedure calls for headlines to be placed on the left, with the story starting to the right, as follows:

```
IF THIS IS              THE STORY CAN START
YOUR HEADLINE           OVER HERE, MOVING
                        OVER TO THE RIGHT
COLUMN, LEAVING ABOUT AN INCH MARGIN, THEN
CONTINUING ON, RETURNING TO THE FULL LEFT-
MARGIN ONCE ENOUGH SPACE HAS BEEN GIVEN TO THE
HEADLINE MAKING IT EASILY LEGIBLE.
```

An alternative calls for centering the headline as follows:

```
            IF THIS IS
           YOUR HEADLINE
    THE STORY WOULD START ABOUT HERE AND
CONTINUE ON WITH THE SAME COLUMN WIDTH IN A
UNIFORM MANNER. THE ONLY PROBLEM WITH THIS
CONCERNS THE CENTERING OF HEADLINES WHICH MAY
COME OUT A LITTLE OFF, AND HENCE LOOK A BIT
AWKWARD.
```

A more complicated style of layout, still using the typewriter, calls for columns, as follows:

```
THE FIRST STORY          IT CAN GET
STARTS HERE              CONFUSING
THE FIRST ARTICLE STARTS USING THIS METHOD CAN
HERE AND PROBABLY WILL   LEAD TO CONFUSION AND
BE CONTINUED ON ANOTHER  CERTAINLY MAKES TYPING
PAGE SOMEWHERE ELSE IN   THE NEWSLETTER A MORE
THE NEWSLETTER.          DIFFICULT JOB.
```

When using the double column method, it is strongly advised to first make up a dummy which shows how the newsletter will be laid out—which article begins where, is continued where, etc. Add additional time for the task.

You also may consider at some time going to typesetting which involves the setting of justified type (perfect margins left and right, like this book). Again, bear in mind that a large size type should be used, 12- or 14-point, to permit easy reading. This will require a complete dummy for use by a typesetter or printer, and adds to expense.

If you elect to use photographs, a dummy should be prepared, regardless of what format is used, to indicate where photos will go, thus enabling the typist to adjust her margins accordingly, or the typesetter to establish runarounds correctly.

Writing

Information on writing is contained in Chapter V. Modification of guidelines for writing a newsletter call for reading of newspapers to see examples of the different style employed in various articles. It is suggested that some stories be bylined (meaning that the name of the author is placed with the article) and that this writer's style be allowed to show itself, rather than being edited into uniformity. In cases of large nursing homes which have a newsletter strictly for outside distribution, a more professional approach may be called for.

Headline Writing

Newspaper have writers on staff who do nothing but prepare headlines. (The headline of a story, even when the story is by-lined, seldom is written by the person writing the story.) If there is someone in your home with a knack for headline writing, enlist his support. A bit of whimsy, when the story is light, is highly desirable.

Name

The publication, of course, should have a distinctive name. An easy, enjoyable method of choosing a name involves the holding of a competition among employees, volunteers and patients. It is suggested that the competition be announced in the first newsletter (which for the time being could be titled THE NO NAME GAZETTE) so readers can get a feeling of what the publication is like before trying to title it.

Standard Format

Once the name of the newsletter is established, you should consider going to a standard front page format, including the name of the newsletter, name and address of the nursing home and similar information. You can select from a variety of different type styles from a typesetter, although it is advised that you utilize either professional or free-lance art talent to get exactly what you want. Once designed and completed, the front page is printed in quantity, and is used as the paper onto which front page copy is printed. If colored paper is used, be certain that the same color paper is used throughout.

Bear in mind that you do not have to use pages stapled together. One can also use a standard 17 x 11-inch format which, when folded vertically down the midle, results in a standard 8½ x 11-inch four-page format. This type format tends to be limiting, however, and can look awkward if not filled, or be inconvenient when more than four pages of copy must be used.

You also may wish to consider developing some type of self-mailing format which will ostensibly eliminate the use of envelopes, except when other material must be enclosed.

Before deciding on any standard format, it is suggested that you contact a state or national nursing home association to see samples of other nursing homes' newsletters, or at least to learn what other homes publish newsletters so you can follow up to obtain samples.

Printing

The selection of a printing method should be based both on cost and appearance criteria, except when patient participation in the printing process is considered essential. In such cases utilization of in-house equipment is advisable. Some of the types of printing available are:

MIMEOGRAPH. Mimeography is economical but sometimes is limiting, especially in cases of long runs where stencils may have to be typed several times. In most cases the quality leaves a lot to be desired. Photos either cannot be used or come out looking very muddy.

XEROGRAPHY. While use of Xerox equipment may not be the least expensive in terms of long runs, it is easy to use and capable of producing good quality. Most models, but not all, do not reproduce photos well.

Itek. This is an inexpensive form of photo offset that usually produces excellent quality at low cost, except that photos cannot be duplicated well.

Photo Offset Printing. Photo offset rapidly is becoming the most popular of nonoffice equipment. It involves photographing the original and making a master plate; not inexpensive, but essential if you want good reproduction of photographs.

A simple savings tip: Use both sides of a sheet of paper when stapled-together sheets are used. It saves on paper and postage costs.

XVIII

MAILING EQUIPMENT

MAILING EQUIPMENT, or at least addressing equipment, is something which all nursing homes should have on hand, for mailing of bills, newsletters, news releases and other materials issued regularly. Actual cost/time savings usually enable mailing/addressing equipment to pay for itself within a few months.

Xerox has a very inexpensive addressing system which comprises a master sheet for typing names, and special pre-cut, gummed-back copying sheets onto which the type names are printed, then peeled off and placed onto envelopes. The problem with this system is the difficulty of making changes, and the waste involved when a mailing is going out only to several portions of those on a master sheet. It also precludes alphabetical listings when, over a period of time, new names are added and others are deleted.

Other systems available are manufactured by, among others, Pitney Bowes and Addressograph-Multigraph. The Pitney Bowes system allows for typing up of plates in your office, while the Addressograph-Multigraph system requires a plate-making machine, or the sending out of names for plates to be made, usually at a cost of 20 to 25 cents per plate. Small, hand-operated Addressograph-Multigraph equipment frequently can be found used for under $50. Larger facilities with very large mailing lists should consider the more automated machines that actually do involve more of the mailing, rather than just addressing functions.

XIX

THE OPEN HOUSE

THE OPEN HOUSE is a frequently-used public relations tool which brings certain publics into the nursing home to inform them of particular information, directly or indirectly.

To be effective, and to avoid any potential backfire, the open house must be thoroughly planned and coordinated. The following guidelines are offered for consideration.

ESTABLISH PURPOSE. You must have a valid reason for holding an open house, not only in your own mind but in the minds of those you invite. If you believe the reason is valid, be certain to phrase your reasoning in terms readily understood and appreciated by those who will be invited.

ESTABLISH PRIME AUDIENCES. You should establish if there are certain publics which are more important than others. If so, consider limiting the open house to just these publics, or to having special hours for prime publics if others are invited as well.

ESTABLISH THE PROGRAM. You must determine what your program will include, planning it in light of the interests of those who will be attending, or those whom you most want to reach. Be sure to consider a guest speaker on the program, or a film (available from an association, for example), or similar program adjuncts, as well as repeating the program at certain times. Be certain that the program is carefully reviewed and rereviewed before committing yourself to it.

TIMING. Be certain that the open house does not conflict with other community activities. If you are concerned about a prime audience, for example, determine what organization or two most audience members belong to and whether or not there will be any major conflicts. By the same token, determine if it would be possible to tie in other activities with your open house. For example, if parishioners of a certain church are a prime audience, could a church service be held in your nursing home as an element of the open house? Also consider what time of day is best for the group involved.

ATTENDANCE. Determine approximately how many people will be attending, and be certain to include patients, employees, volunteers, patient families and friends, state and local officials and others. It is better to plan for too many than for not enough.

SPECIAL ENTERTAINMENT. If you do intend to provide some sort of special entertainment, be certain it is appropriate for the public (s) involved and the purpose of the open house.

CONDITION OF THE HOME. Make a thorough check of the home prior to having an open house. If there is some touch-up work to be done, be certain that it can and will be done prior to the open house. If it cannot be done in time, consider rescheduling the open house.

DECORATIONS. If the open house will be built on a theme, such as a national theme, Christmas theme, etc., it may be very worthwhile to decorate the home accordingly. Be certain to determine who will be in charge of decorating; making and obtaining decorations; when work will begin on decorating, etc. Such activities usually can be tied in with a patient activities program.

TOURS. You may wish to have tours of the home and its grounds as part of your open house. Determine what the tour route shall be, including first stop, second stop, and so forth; who will lead tour groups; what will be said at each stop; whether any disruption of routine will be caused and, if so, what can be done to compensate for it.

INVITATIONS. Determine who will be in charge of invitations and how they shall be issued, as through advertising, news release, phone, letter or personal encounter; whether or not it will be RSVP; who will prepare a list of names and how, and related concerns.

RECEPTION AREA. Determine what area will be used as a reception area and whether or not furniture will have to be rearranged, clothes racks rented, and so forth. Plan logistics in advance to eliminate as much last minute confusion as possible.

WRITTEN PROGRAM. If there are a variety of events to be undertaken, consider making up a written program for the participants as well as visitors. Be certain to have it written and printed well ahead of time.

SPECIAL EQUIPMENT. Determine what special equipment, if any, will be necessary and plan to arrange for it ahead of time. Such equipment could include extra chairs, tables, coat racks, punch bowls, cups, etc., as well as projectors (slide? film strip? 8 MM? Super 8? 16 MM? Sound?), microphones, amplifiers, movie screens, a podium, extension cords, easel, chalkboard and chalk, etc. By all means have at least one sign-in guest book, writing implements and possibly a stand or podium.

PHOTOGRAPHY. Be certain that either an "in-house" or professional photographer will be on hand. Be prepared to make prints for news releases, for the scrapbook and photo library, as well as for souvenir photos to be sent to several of those who attend.

PRESS RELATIONS. Assign responsibilities for press relations. A news release should be sent out prior to the open house, if appropriate, as well as after. If celebrities, such as congressmen, are to be on hand, and if they are to present a talk of some sort, a draft of the talk or at least its subject should be obtained for distribution to news media. Determine which members of the press, if any, should be invited.

PATIENT COORDINATION. Someone must be appointed to coordinate activities with patients, preparing them for the open house. It may require extra personnel in the fields of hair dressing and grooming if all patients are to look their best at the same time. Obviously, since the nursing home is the patients' home and community, they should be involved in as many open house activities as possible.

REFRESHMENTS. Determine what type refreshments are appropriate, and bear in mind that it may be necessary to have personnel on hand to ensure that patients with dietary restrictions do not partake of those foods which could be harmful. Be certain, in such cases, that special refreshments are available for those who require them.

PARKING. Parking can be a serious problem unless carefully planned. Determine who will be responsible for showing people where to park, and that all necessary permits for parking will be taken care of. The local police department may be able to help if required. Also, determine if special insurance may be necessary.

ROOM CHANGES. Determine if certain rooms or areas will have to be converted from one use to another during the open house. If so, be certain to assign personnel to handle such tasks. It may be best to hold a trial run beforehand to ensure that everyone knows where certain things go, and when they go there.

PERSONNEL ON HAND. Determine beforehand which personnel must be in attendance, as well as what should be done regarding uniforms and related concerns. Also consider who will be on vacation at the time of the open house as well as how much overtime pay is involved.

GREETERS. Several staff members should be assigned to greet and orient people as they arrive. Those who have such tasks should be attractive, glib, and easily able to communicate. Be certain to check timetables to ensure that greeters will be on hand at all times.

TOUR DIRECTORS. Be certain that tour directors are fully acquainted with the tour route and what they will be saying in regard to certain elements of the tour. Also, be certain that they are aware of all relevant safety and fire safety rules.

LEGAL CONSIDERATIONS. Determine if there are any legal considerations you may have overlooked, such as the number of persons who may be in a certain room at a certain time.

LITERATURE. Ascertain what literature you would like to hand out to visitors, such as brochures on the home itself, nursing homes in general, magazine article reprints, etc. Be certain that orders are placed well enough in advance to have on hand everything you wish to distribute.

RAIN. Be prepared for the worst in regard to the weather. Have alternative action plans developed in case outdoor activities are planned.

Rain usually means more automobiles and more outergarments.

CLEAN UP. Be certain that clean-up plans are included in general planning. Determine who will be assigned to clean-up efforts and how long it will take so you can estimate when the routine will be returning to normal, and what interim plans must be put in effect until they are.

THANK-YOUS. Make arrangements for thanking all those who attended either through written letters, telephone calls, etc.

Bear in mind that the above listing is partial, but it can be used as a basis, and will suggest other considerations in and of itself. The key fact to remember is this: You are inviting into your nursing home many people, each of whom will be forming opinions based mostly on what he sees and hears. If you do not plan well, you are relinquishing control and so inviting the unexpected to occur, thereby jeopardizing achievement of goals, and possibly creating a bad image where a good one or at least none existed before.

XX

PAID ADVERTISING

WHILE RELATIVELY FEW nursing homes find it necessary to advertise, it is an essential for those homes which are opening new or expanded facilities; which have a large vacancy rate, or which attempt to rely primarily on private patients.

Depending on the expense which you intend to budget for advertising or on the length of time which you intend to devote to a campaign, it may or may not be practical to hire an advertising agency. For example, if the advertising is to be put into effect only for a short period of time, and if the budget is small, the assistance which the medium is able to provide may be sufficient. If a lengthy, costly program is anticipated, however, you should seek the guidance of a competent advertising agency.

Selecting an Advertising Agency

Because of the large amounts of money which can be spent in an advertising campaign, it is imperative that your selection be made with deliberate care. The following guidelines should stand you in good stead:

MAKE A LIST. Prepare a listing of advertising agencies by seeking references from business acquaintances, by using the Yellow Pages, or by asking a local newspaper advertising account executive for a listing of seven or eight reliable agencies. Also if you see or hear an ad which you feel is particularly good, call the advertiser to determine who prepared it.

CONTACT THE AGENCIES. Ask an account executive of each listed agency to forward some materials concerning his agency. Typical materials include a brochure, listing of clients, case histories and resumes.

NARROW DOWN THE LIST. Examine the material supplied by the various firms and determine which, in your opinion, are most competent in terms of general experience, experience with health care facilities, success of previous campaigns, and related matters. List the top three firms in order of preference.

CONTACT EACH OF THREE FIRMS. Contact representatives of the three firms one at a time, going over the manner in which they feel your needs can be filled, what media should be used, and the costs involved, other than costs for space or time purchased. Determine if the firm will use a retainer arrangement, rather than commission, so you pay only for time and materials involved, plus net cost of space (less commission). By use of this method, rather than straight commission, the agency does not get into a position of suggesting purchase of time or space primarily to increase commissionable revenues.

SELECT A FIRM. Determine which firm you want to use on the basis of value, realizing that the lowest cost does not necessarily mean the best value.

Determining the Medium

One of the most critical elements in advertising is determination of the media to utilize. Several criteria should be considered.

ACTUAL MARKET. Let us assume that paper A has a readership of 100,000 and paper B has a readership of 200,000. An ad in paper A cost $100, the same ad in paper B costing $150. On the surface, it would appear that paper B is clearly the better buy. But is it? To determine which paper offers the most value, first determine who comprises the readership of each paper. If paper A's readership includes 10,000 persons aged 50 or more, who would have parents possibly in need of nursing home care, and paper B also has 10,000, clearly the size of prime target publics are the same and thus paper A is the better buy. In other words, what you are interested in is the size of your market which the medium reaches, not the total number of people reached.

POSITION. It also is important to know which paper or medium gives the best time slot or position. In a newspaper, for example, if you can get the exact position you prefer, without extra cost, it can mean increased readership without additional expense. Now let's go back to our example above, with like amounts of potential patients or patient families. If paper A places your ad in a bad position, perhaps only 25 percent of your prime target public will read it. If paper B gives you the position you prefer, perhaps up to 80 percent of your market will read your ad and, in that case, paper B clearly becomes the better buy. The same applies to radio. A so-called bargain becomes a waste of money if your ad is aired at three o'clock in the morning.

Media Considerations

There are a variety of media appropriate for your advertising. Some comments on each appear below.

NEWSPAPERS, DAILY. Daily newspapers by and large are the largest in the area. As for all media, be concerned with certain vital statistics, such as: the number of subscribers and total newsstand sales; amount of readers (readership is always more than sales) and their age, location and sex. Bear in mind that newsstand sales often mean readership by a male at the office or during lunch, whereas home delivery usually indicates readership by the family, husband and wife.

NEWSPAPERS, WEEKLY. Weekly newspapers are published once a week and are delivered or mailed to the home. Usually they are sent to a particular area, and often do not have the mass readership of a daily paper. Be certain to determine what type weekly is involved. For example, many weekly newspapers are geared primarily for classified advertising copy. As a result, display advertising, that advertising which appears intermingled with news sections and not under a certain classification, may not have as much impact, most readers being concerned strictly with classified headings.

RADIO. Radio is an exceptionally effective medium in that it reaches a particular type audience, as compared to a newspaper which attracts a general audience, or an audience whose only commonality is location. For example, you can easily tell that a radio station which plays semiclassical music and sounds of the Big Bands probably has a prime listenership aged forty or more. On the other hand, a station which plays primarily "hard rock" appeals mostly to youth. Radio stations usually can provide demographic data, and you can easily measure the potential market each station reaches.

TELEVISION. Television reaches a mass audience of all ages and is relatively inexpensive in terms of cost per thousand people reached. However, because most of each dollar spent will go to reaching viewers who rarely are interested in nursing home care, it is not a recommended medium.

YELLOW PAGES. Yellow Pages advertising can be very costly. If the competition in your area is slight, a bold faced heading may be all that is needed. Conversely, heavy competition may require more extensive advertising, such as in-column advertising, or display space. The author's experience has been that in-column advertising yields the most value from each Yellow Pages advertising dollar. In pricing Yellow Pages advertising, remember to determine what the costs will be for the year.

MAGAZINES. Investigate whatever magazines are published in your area, considering demographic statistics and availability of preferred positioning. Advertising in magazines or related periodicals which are associated primarily with charitable or civic organizations should be considered donations. Do not expect significant returns.

OTHER. There are many other types of advertising available, including billboards, bumper strips, etc. Bear in mind that where you advertise as well as the way you advertise has much to do with development of your image. For example, advertising on a bowling lane score sheet is hardly appropriate for the type services which you offer.

Advertising Content

Determining what to say in your advertisement is basically a matter left up to you. As a general rule, consider the value of establishing credibility and reliability with the audience. Mention the licenses, memberships (as in ANHA or AAHA), and accreditations which you have and key personnel have earned. Above all, be truthful in your advertising. If graphic elements are involved, be certain that any representations of the home itself are accurate. Do not try to create an image of a tree-lined driveway if the trees do not exist. The image you strive to develop must be an accurate reflection of what actually exists. If it is not, whatever image you attempt to establish will backfire in the face of truth and so defeat the entire purpose of your endeavors.

In cases where you determine not to utilize an advertising agency, bear in mind that each medium usually has a staff which can assist you in preparation of copy, design and other elements at little or no charge.

General Program

There are several ways of establishing a general program. One school of thought favors utilizing one medium at a time, while the other favors a concurrent combination of media so that each can reinforce the other. If your advertising is geared primarily for the short term, a multiple approach is best, keeping copy for a newspaper ad almost identical to copy for a radio ad, thereby creating close identification betwen the two. In this way, people are most apt to connect the two and remember the advertiser, rather than thinking of them as represening two different organizations.

Some Insider's Tips

A few tips to consider are these:

RADIO. Try to get a package deal. Most stations will give them whether or not they are on the rate card. A good package usually entails a variety of spots, a certain amount within each given time period, AM Drive, 10-4 PM drive, early evening, late evening. When possible, specify which hours within each time segment you want your ads to air. Another possibility is an ROS (Run of the Station) package, which means your ads will air whenever the station has time available. This usually is the least expensive plan available, for obvious reasons. If you buy ROS, be certain to specify when you would like your spots to air. Be aware that many radio stations will prepare a rate card which is far removed from the price which they will accept. Oftentimes $20 per minute spots will sell for $12. In addition, if you do not utilize an agency, realize that the station usually is saving the 15 percent an agency normally receives in commission.

NEWSPAPERS. Newspapers usually work on a contract basis. If you agree to purchase 10,000 lines in a year, you receive a much better rate than if you advertise without a contract (open rate). Similarly, you pay far less per line with a 100,000-line rate than you do with a 10,000-line rate. Typically, the paper makes a tally at year's end to determine how much space you have used. If you have used more than you contracted for, and have gone to the next higher contract, you will get credit or rebate. If you have used less than contracted, you will get a bill on the basis of the contract which should have been in force. Therefore, if you plan a somewhat lengthy campaign, it is advised to utilize a contract much larger than anticipated (if the paper will accept this) and pay the difference at year's end, more or less using the paper's money rather than having the paper use yours. Also, in ordering print media advertising, be certain to specify what position you would like to have. Often you receive it at no extra cost.

XXI

PUBLIC SERVICE
ADVERTISING

PUBLIC SERVICE ADVERTISING is a frequently overlooked element
of public relations which can provide handsome rewards for
those who utilize it. It requires the nursing home either to offer
something to the community as a public service, or to request a
public service of the community. Broadcast media in particular
like public service advertising because they must air a certain
amount of such advertising as part of their responsibilities and
requirements for holding a broadcast license. Newspapers and
other print media also will utilize such advertising, although usually not to such an extent.

Possible Programs

Public service advertising is not a gimmick. You must have
either a legitimate offer of public service or a legitimate public
service request or, as in many cases, offer a program which is a
two-way street, enabling the nursing home to do something for
the community and the community to do something for patients
and themselves. For example, having an exhibition of arts and
crafts made by patients would be an excellent item for public
service advertising, advising community members that they can
see what patients have made, and in so doing enjoy themselves and
bring joy to patients. A request for persons to staff up a volunteer
program would emphasize patients' needs for outside community
involvement, while also stressing that community members would
have a wonderful way to serve their fellow man. You may wish to
undertake the offering of a program instructing participants in
home care for the aged, involving three or four evening seminars
in your dining or community room, with talks given by yourself
and certain staff members, including subjects of cooking, mobility,

safety, etc. This course would cost you little; would be readily accepted for public service advertising time and, of course, would win recognition for the nursing home, particularly on the part of those attending the courses. Another possibility would be the offering of a booklet or booklets regarding selection of a nursing home free to those who send in or come in for the information. (You can obtain a supply from the government and/or American Nursing Home Association.) The possibilities are limited only by your own imagination.

Preparing a Public Service Ad

To prepare the advertisement itself, first get together all pertinent facts, answering questions who, what, when, where, how and why. Your advertising agency or PR firm should be able to develop appropriate materials or, if you do not use such firms, the media themselves often will be happy to help, although you should offer to at least underwrite expenses involved. In either case, before any advertising is prepared, be certain to visit the advertising directors of the various local media *in person* to discuss the idea and the medium's requirements and, where applicable, to deliver copy, photographs, and other materials.

To give you an idea of what is entailed, consider the following radio copy:

> Are you thinking about a nursing home for yourself, a friend or relative? If so, be sure you know what's involved before making any decision, because selection of a nursing home is vitally important to the health and well-being of those who require long-term care. To provide you with information, the XYZ Nursing Home has available at no charge several booklets prepared by the federal government and the American Nursing Home Association. To obtain copies of these brochures, either come to the home or write. The address is. . . .

For television, the exact same copy can be used accompanied either by slides of nursing home activity and the booklets, or by motion picture footage shot by the TV station itself. For print media, the same copy can be used accompanied by a photograph of the booklets or a typical nursing home scene.

Bear in mind that any program worthy of public service advertising also is worthy of a news release. In the case of the free brochure, for example, a news release issued at the beginning of the program would indicate availability, using much the same copy as in the advertising, while another release several weeks later would indicate the results of the program, announcing that 1000 or so booklets had been distributed.

Be certain to send thanks to those advertising directors who give you public service time or space.

XXII

GREETING CARDS

PERHAPS ONE OF THE simplest of all PR programs to operate involves the mailing of greeting cards to various individuals on birthdays, religious and lay holidays, and other occasions. While certainly not a program designed to establish good will in and of itself, it can help improve good will when used in conjunction with other programs, and definitely can help maintain contact with a variety of persons affiliated and unaffiliated with the home.

Establish a List

The first step in establishing the program is to create a list of occasions and persons who should be remembered, including:

BIRTHDAYS. For all patients, employees and volunteers, whose birth dates can be ascertained from records. Also, various officials and others whose birthdays you learn. A calendar can be made up near the end of the year for use in the next year which shows who will be having a birthday when. All patients should be sent birthday cards, but those sent to others, such as employees, should be sent only when the employee is known on sight. If you do not take the time to learn an employee's name and talk with him, but do send him a birthday greeting, chances are the card approach will backfire, and will be seen as little more than a sham.

HOLIDAYS. Such as Valentine's Day (especially for female patients, employees, volunteers, and others, providing the administrator is male); St. Patrick's Day (primarily for those of Irish ancestry); Easter (mostly for those of Catholic faith); Rosh Hashanah (for those of Jewish faith); Christmas and New Year's, or "Season's Greetings," for just about everybody. Naturally, other holidays can be added should you wish.

OTHER OCCASIONS. Requiring get well, sympathy and other type cards.

Sending

In sending cards, which can be purchased in quantity, care should be taken to at least sign each one (either personally or have someone do it for you), or to add a personal note. Envelopes should be hand addressed.

XXIII

PUBLIC SPEAKING

PUBLIC SPEAKING IS a very effective communications tool which can be made into an important element of an overall public relations program. While many of the techniques of person-to-person interpersonal communications are applicable to public speaking, you are reaching a much larger audience and are in a semi-authoritative position. If you believe in what you are talking about, you can far more easily convince the public listening to you of your own sincerity, and so maximize potential support of your message.

The biggest drawback to public speaking is fear. It is something which many have never been called upon to do, and hence they regard it with some degree of fright, perhaps masked by skepticism of its possible benefits. The facts of the matter are these: public speaking itself is not difficult, nor is it difficult to obtain speaking engagements or prepare a talk. And even if these tasks were difficult, the benefits which can be obtained would make the effort worthwhile.

Possible Subjects

As in all PR programming, any message delivered first must be geared to the audience involved. The subject of nursing homes, because each nursing home is a self-contained community within a community at-large, is not difficult. In many cases, the audience simply will be interested in knowing what a nursing home really is like and what it does. But more often, they will be interested in their particular aspect. For example, a garden club would be interested in knowing the benefits of indoor and outdoor gardening for the nursing home patient, and possibly how they can help in a program of gardening in the context of occupational therapy or activities programming. Jaycees would be interested in knowing how certain patients in your nursing home have contributed to the community in the past; how they still can contribute, and perhaps how the Jaycees can become involved in home activities. Members of the Chamber of Commerce or Better Business Bureau would be concerned about the nursing home industry as a whole, what is being done to upgrade, and how your home attempts to develop quality programming. High school or college students would want to know about possible careers in health care and nursing homes, what training is involved, how advancement is made, etc. Women's and civic organizations probably would be interested in volunteering in nursing homes and how community volunteers, as friendly visitors or as elements of an overall volunteer or activities program, can contribute meaningfully to the lives of patients and to their own lives. Business groups may be interested in the economics of nursing homes. Health care personnel may want to know about special programs for nursing home patients, new development in geriatric care, and related facts. And so the list goes on, more or less basing the subject on the audience involved, thereby making the talk relevant.

Each time a talk is given, the speaker is seen by the audience as an authority in the field, and the nursing home he represents as exemplary, a benefit to the community, and the most likely choice should a nursing home be needed.

Obtaining Material

It is relatively easy to obtain material on any given subject, and it is advised that development of a speaker's library be begun in your home even before activities toward obtaining speaking engagements are undertaken. Material for talks can be obtained from prepared speeches available from state and national associations; texts of speeches of national associations' and other groups' officers; from newspaper and magazine articles and informational brochures and, of course, from one's own experience. An effort should be made to clip, save and file material by subject so, once a speaker's program begins, it will be a relatively simple matter to prepare a talk.

Obtaining Speaking Engagements

The first step in obtaining speaking engagements is to list the various organizations in your community including business and civic organizations, fraternal orders, women's clubs, and so forth. Very often a Chamber of Commerce has such a list. In other cases a survey of employees and volunteers can be made asking them about organizations which they and their family know of.

The second step is to develop a list of contacts. In some cases you will belong to some of the organizations listed. In other cases friends or other contacts belong. It may even be necessary to ask friends of friends, until contact is made, and the name of an organization's president or program committee chairman is learned.

The third step is to make contact and make known your availability as a speaker, first, of course, determining what you will talk about. It is advised that you start on the most friendly territory first, such as organizations you belong to, or those in which friends hold office. With other groups, simply contact the appropriate individual in person, or by phone or letter, and state that you would like to speak before the group if they do on occasion have guest speakers. In cases where speaking programs are booked solid, find out when an appropriate time would be to make application to deliver a talk during the next year.

Finalizing Arrangements

Once you do get a speaking engagement, be certain to finalize arrangements. This includes knowing exactly where and when the talk is to be given, how much time should be taken, whether or not a question-answer session will follow, whether or not you can distribute materials, etc. Also, you should inform the organization about your needs, including a microphone, podium (if you have notes), a light (for reading the speech if you are not familiar enough with it to work from memory or hand-held cards), projection equipment, easel, and so forth.

Preparing the Talk

It has been said that, when delivering a talk, one should tell the audience what you are about to tell them; tell them; then tell them what you told them. In essence, this means introduction, main material, summary. For the most part, you can follow instructions given in Chapter V on writing and, especially, organizing. One key point to bear in mind is this: written English and spoken English are almost two different languages. Therefore, once you write your talk, it is imperative to read it aloud and make all changes necessary to make the talk a talk, and not just a reading of a written document. More specifically, follow these guidelines when preparing a talk from scratch, or personalizing a model:

DON'T USE BIG WORDS. A "big word" does not have to be long and polysyllabic, but very often it is. Many people like to use big words because they're convinced it shows listeners how educated they are. But that isn't what the audience came to find out. To be sure that your audience understands what you're talking about, use as many commonplace words as possible: No "albeit" and "wherefore" when "but" and "why" will do; don't "disseminate information" when you can just "give the facts." If you have to use terms germane to the profession, explain them first—in detail.

KEEP SENTENCES SHORT. When writing a document, long sentences are sometimes acceptable. One can always hunt back to find the verb, subject, etc. But one cannot hunt when listening to a talk. Keep the sentences short and clear. If an audience has to figure out what you just said, it means they've totally lost what you're saying now.

REMENTION WHAT YOU'RE REFERRING TO. If you have to refer back to something, avoid "it," "which," "who," etc., because it may only tend to confuse the audience. Do not be afraid to remention names or statistics. Written out it may look foolish, but a live audience will appreciate it. If you are dealing with a variety of different names and/or statistics, so that even rementioning may become confusing, it may be best to use an easel and some handwritten charts, just to ensure that the audience is with you all the way.

USE VISUALS WHEN APPROPRIATE. Visuals, such as slides of photos you may have on file, nearly always add interest to your talk. If you are going to use slides throughout your talk, as opposed to using them just during certain segments, be sure you have enough on hand to prevent one slide from being on screen for too long.

BE SPECIFIC ABOUT AN ACTION REQUEST. If you ask your audience to do something, be specific about your request without "pussyfooting." For example, "Those are the statistics. So I want each one of you to sign this petition now to avoid what easily could be a calamity for this community."

LOCALIZE FACTS. Many prepared speeches will come with facts pertaining to the nation. To heighten audience interest, include or substitute related statistics pertinent to your region, state or community.

SUM UP WITHOUT SUMMING UP. The last point made in your speech should sum up, in as few words as possible, the entirety of what you've said. To emphasize the point, don't clutter it up with "And in conclusion," "In summation," or similar phrases. Make it a hard-hitting declarative sentence, such as: "The nursing home—a community within a community. A place designed to help its patients retain and regain as great a degree of self-reliance and self-respect as possible." (Compare with, "And in conclusion, I think you can see that the nursing home really is a community within a community, where we sincerely try to help patients retain and regain their abilities in many different areas.")

Delivering Your Talk

The manner in which a speech is delivered is important. If it's too smooth, it can make your audience feel as though you do not necessarily believe in what you are saying. If it's too ragged, even the most powerful talk can turn into a confusing mess. For best results, keep in mind the following brief guidelines.

TYPE THE SPEECH. Ideally you should be able to deliver your talk without use of notes of any kind. If you are not familiar enough with it to do that, however, the second best method is to use 3 x 5 note cards with key words written on each. If you are not familiar enough with the talk to do that, then by all means type the speech so you can avoid mistakes.

When typing, use an IBM Orator font if you have an IBM Selectric typewriter available. Otherwise, use all capital letters and triple space, making it easy to find your place when looking back to the page after looking up at the audience. Do not end a line with a hyphenated word. Do not end a page in the middle of a paragraph. Indicate emphasis by underlining in red or by leaving space between words. For example: WE CAN, AND WE SHALL MAKE THIS COMMUNITY A BETTER PLACE TO LIVE.

BE AS FAMILIAR WITH THE SPEECH AS POSSIBLE. Even though you may have to use the typed speech before the audience, be familiar with it so you can look up at the audience as much as possible. Familiarize yourself with the speech by reading it aloud at least seven times. Read it before your family or others and ask for frank criticism. Also, read it before a mirror and tape record what you've said. Listen to the recording critically and, if there are parts of the speech you wish to change or emphasize, make markings on the typed pages for your reference while speaking.

DON'T BE LIFELESS. When you are before your audience, do not act like an automaton, merely standing there and reading. Put life into your talk. Move around on the podium. Mention names of people in the audience when appropriate. Talk to the audience, rather than lecture them.

DON'T SAY "UH!"

Ad-Libbing

To ad-lib, according to Webster, means to "deliver spontaneously." This means that your ad-libs, and they do help to emphasize a point or to insert some comic relief if it's needed, should be delivered in a casual manner and cannot be read.

BE FAMILIAR WITH YOUR AD-LIB (s). Know the story well before attempting to tell it, and be sure it is germane to the topic being discussed at the time of its introduction. Merely indicate an ad-lib in the following manner: THAT OCCURRED IN 1970, AND IT REMINDS ME OF A STORY. *AFTER AD LIB COME IN HERE:* SO YOU SEE, NONE OF US IS

USE AD-LIBS SPARINGINGLY. Remember that even when used to emphasize a point, an ad-lib is a digression, and as such a sidetrack. The more you use, the more sidetracked your talk becomes. Use ad-libs sparingly, however, and they can help balance your talk and make it far more enjoyable for all concerned. Be sure each ad-lib is relevant. Be sure you are familiar with each one.

Some PR Considerations

While public speaking in and of itself is an excellent PR tool, as already mentioned, it can be made even more worthwhile through several gambits.

PRESS RELEASES. Determine a month or so prior to the talk if the group before which you shall speak has PR staff or PR capabilities. If not, you should handle issuing press releases. Regardless of who assumes the responsibility, the following should be done:

Issue a press release prior to the talk, including a photograph of the speaker with caption. The release should detail when and where the talk will be given, whether or not the public is invited, how to make reservations, etc. Be sure to time the release effectively, especially for weekly papers which should have the release in time to publish it before the talk is given.

Invite the press, if appropriate, by contacting appropriate editors several days prior to sending out the release. For weekly papers, an invitation to the editor-in-chief is correct. For dailies, choose the editor most appropriate, Food Editor, Garden Editor, or what-have-you.

Issue a press release following the talk, based primarily on a summary of the speech text. A photo also should accompany this release. The release should be mailed out prior to the talk for weeklies, so it will be published immediately after the talk, and the day of the talk to dailies.

Address Texts. Just as reprints of magazine articles are excellent vehicles for establishing you as an authority in your field in the eyes of those who did not read the article when it was published in a magazine, so does the text of a speech, edited, set in type and printed, help to establish you as an authority in the eyes of those who did not hear your talk. To have the text printed, first edit it or have it edited, and bring it to the printer who should use large bold type across the top of an 8½ x 11 inch page to indicate the title of the talk and in italics below that, "Text of an address delivered before the (name of the group, date), by (name, title). The text can be set in ten-point type, such as century schoolbook, double columned. Have the material printed on quality, enamel stock, and distribute and use just as you would a magazine reprint.

XXIV

MAGAZINE ARTICLES

W^{E LIVE TODAY} in what has been titled a "diploma-oriented" society. For one reason or another we tend to evaluate a person not by what he can do, but rather by what he has done. For example, given two equally qualified persons applying for the same job, except only one has a master's degree, the job probably will go to the one with the master's degree. Similarly, given fifty nursing home administrators about equal in terms of knowledge and experience, the one regarded as the authority in the field will be the one who has written the most on the subject of nursing homes and nursing home administration. In fact, what a person has done in terms of writing about a subject sometimes supercedes his education. Going back to the first example, had the applicant without the master's written several authorative articles on a relevant subject, published in good trade magazines, chances are he would have been the one hired.

What we are saying, in essence, is this: The faults of judging people by what they have done and not by what they can do work only against those who have done very little.

Accordingly, one of the fastest and easiest ways to work with the system is to write and submit articles for publication.

The basic criteria of any article must be that it has something meaningful to say. As simple as this may sound, it often is a bugaboo for those completely involved in what they are doing. For example, development of a new activities program in your nursing home may seem to be nothing of any major consequence to you, but for others just beginning such a program, the experience you detail could have tremendous impact. Therefore, you must strive to be somewhat objective about who you are, what you do, and what is being done in your nursing home, to really determine what is worthwhile.

To determine what subjects are good for what type publications, merely read publications to see what type articles are being published. Consider magazines concerned only with nursing homes, as well as those dealing with geriatric care, health care in general, hospitals, and so forth. Chances are many of the stories appearing in such publications will give you ideas of your own. And do not forget other specialized publications for which you can make your subject appropriate, just as discussed in Chapter XXIII. As an example, a publication on gardening probably would be interested in an article on gardening's positive effects on nursing home patients. A magazine on dietary matters may be interested in a discussion of special diets for special illnesses. And so the list goes on. The important point to remember is this: Having your name in print as the author of an article dealing with a subject in which you are involved reflects excellently on yourself and, of course, on your nursing home. It establishes you as an authority on your subject, and one whose opinions should be trusted. Moreover, the positive value of having articles published far exceed whatever cost is necessary in terms of time or expense for editorial assistance. And even editorial costs may be eliminated if a magazine's editor lends a hand, or if payment for the article is sufficient to defray costs of professional assistance.

Writing the Article

For the most part, writing instructions given in Chapter V will suffice for magazine article writing, with some slight additions. In many cases you will find it worthwhile to begin a story with an interesting anecdote which relates directly to the heart of your article and what you have to say. It creates immediate reader interest and can serve as an example for later use. Reading of a variety of magazine articles will illustrate this technique, but realize that it may not be necessary for all articles, nor appropriate. Above all, remember that if what you have to say is worthwhile, editorial staff at the magazine probably will give you a hand. So do not let lack of your own or available ability deter you.

Submitting a Story Outline

In some cases you may wish to first develop your article in outline form and submit it in that manner to a magazine editor (his name and address usually is listed in the front of a magazine). A letter should accompany the article stating why you think it is relevant for the magazine involved, what key points will be made, about how many words you think it will be, and your own background and related information, also asking if there is interest. Send only one such letter and outline to a magazine at one time. If you receive back a negative reply, or if you have received no reply within four weeks and have in the interim sent a second letter to which you have not received a reply, try another magazine. If you exhaust all your possible outlets, either do not write the article or write it and have it printed yourself, as discussed below.

Submitting an Article

TYPING. When typing the article in its final form:
Use 8½ x 11 inch paper;
be sure the type is clean;
leave wide margins on either side;
double space;
number pages, and;
put your name on the top of each page.

SENDING. When sending the article into the magazine editor without first submitting a story outline:
Include a brief note explaining why you wrote the article and why you feel it is important;
send the original of the article, and keep a copy for yourself;
include a stamped, self-addressed return envelope in case the article is not deemed satisfactory;
submit to only one magazine at one time, and;
where possible, submit photos with captions, making sure that you have photographic releases and indicating that fact to the editor. If you do not have photos, but can take them if the editor so desires, then by all means inform him that photos will be available if desired.

INQUIRING. After four week's time, if you have not had a reply, write a letter inquiring if the material arrived and, if so, when you will hear word of whether or not it is acceptable.

If the Article is Accepted

If the article is accepted, be certain to purchase ten or so copies of the entire magazine for your own purposes. Inquire as to the cost of having reprints of the article made up by the magazine, and also inquire of a local printer how much reprints would cost printed on enamel stock. Your local printer probably can supply them for less than the magazine. When doing your own reprinting, be certain to check with the magazine regarding a statement stating, "Reprinted from. . . ."

DISTRIBUTING. Distribute copies of the article to families of patients and others. This often can be done in business letters with a P.S. stating, "Enclosed please find a reprint of a recent article which I felt you might find of interest." Copies should be placed in a reception area, or given to families of prospective patients.

AFTERUSE. Bear in mind that a good article easily can be rewritten for another publication, perhaps directed at a different audience. It also can serve as the basis of a speech.

If the Article is Not Accepted

If the article is not accepted on the first try, resubmit to another magazine, rewriting if necessary. If you cannot get the article published, do not be discouraged. Begin another. At the same time, if you feel that the article is well-written, and its major drawback is that magazines already have covered the same material in depth, simply print the article yourself, following the format of any trade magazine you like, without, of course, using its name.

XXV

COMPLAINT HANDLING MECHANISM

THE WAY IN which you handle complaints, and the results obtained from your procedures, are an ultimate test of your public relations capabilities. To an extent, everyone with a complaint is a potential enemy, and it is up to you to resolve the issue and by so doing at least neutralize anger, without creating animosity in other quarters.

The correct handling of complaints involves establishment of a set procedure for all employees to follow. In fact, it would not at all be amiss to include pertinent instructions for employees in the employee handbook, as well as advice on whom to see regarding complaints in the patient policy handbook.

The following guidelines are suggested for use.

If the Complaint is Made in Person

If the complaint is made in person, employees should be informed to immediately call on the administrator or his assistant or deputy.

If the administrator or his representative is not in:

1. A secretary or some other competent member of staff should allow the complainant to do all the talking while she takes down notes, relating to the nature of the complaint, what dates and persons were involved, and as many other facts as possible. She also should obtain the person's name, address and home and business telephone numbers.

2. The information should be given immediately to whomever is designated as having authority to deal with complaints.

3. The persons in authority should review the material as soon as possible and call the person with the complaint to review circumstances and obtain more facts. Genuine concern must be evidenced.

4. As soon as possible, the complaint must be investigated, and handled as discussed below.

NOTE WELL: In no case should a standard form be prepared for recording complaints. It merely indicates that complaints come in so frequently that a form has to be made to handle them all. Also, a form is very cold and impersonal, and often will serve only to aggravate the situation. Further, no instructions should be given regarding the ordering of questions, a secretary going through a fill-in-the-blanks type procedure. This has the same negative effects as a form, and impedes a person with a complaint from getting it off his chest which, in some cases, is a cathartic action in and of itself.

When the administrator or his representative is in:

1. The person with the complaint should be taken into the office as soon as possible.

2. The nursing home staff representative should introduce himself and offer a cup of coffee or tea.

3. The staffer should ask about the nature of the complaint, taking down notes regarding pertinent facts and associated items.

4. Once the person with the complaint has given all the information, the staffer should read it back, making sure that all facts are recorded correctly.

5. If feasible, investigation should begin immediately. If it is a mistake in billing, you may be able to take the complaint directly to the billing department for review of records.

If the complaint involves a misunderstanding regarding charges, or a misunderstanding which somehow involves communication, materials which the person with the complaint was given (and should have read) should be produced and reviewed. (Bear in mind that it may be easiest to advise simply that a misunderstanding must have resulted because your method of communicating was not effective enough, and make adjustments accordingly.) If the complaint involves actions of personnel, locate those involved by *personally* finding them and discussing the situation on the way back to the office. Have those involved in the complaint confront the person making the complaint, yourself acting as mediator. When the situation is discussed fully, employees should be dismissed, being told that you will contact them shortly, which, of course, you should do.

Whenever possible, try to resolve the situation quickly. If the employee is at fault, make necessary apologies and take remedial actions. If it appears that the employee definitely is not at fault, explain the situation to the complainant. If there is doubt in your mind inform the complainant that further investigation is required, and you will be back in touch. Get back in touch as soon as possible, within a day or so, by telephone, or by personal visit, followed by a letter. Be certain to inform employees involved of what is happening.

If the persons involved are not on duty at the time the complaint is registered, follow up as described above, as quickly and accurately as possible.

NOTE WELL: In cases where a law suit may be involved, be certain not to say or to put into writing anything before consulting your attorney.

If the Complaint is Telephoned in:

If the complaint comes via telephone, it should be transferred to someone in authority immediately.

If no one is in, a secretary should take down the information as suggested above. Before contacting the complainant, some basic research should be performed, and the complainant should be invited to come in in person. If he chooses not to come in, follow the procedures suggested above by telephone, being certain to act as quickly as possible. *If the call can be transferred,* act quickly. The nature of the complaint and associated information should be written down and read back for review. The complainant should be advised that research will begin immediately and that he will be called back within a half-hour. At the end of a half-hour, regardless of how research is coming along, he should be called back to be told what progress is being made. Once all facts are known, he should be called again, or be invited to come in in person for discussion, the outcome to be followed by a letter, providing no legal action seems to be involved.

If the Complaint is Written

If the complaint is in writing, immediate research should begin with the complainant being called as soon as possible to discuss the overall situation. A follow-up letter is advised providing legal questions are not involved.

If the Complaint is Made by a Patient

In cases where a patient makes a complaint directly to administration, it should be reviewed immediately and, where possible, the situation should be resolved. If it is a matter of phantom complaints, made and remade primarily to gain sympathy or extra attention, those responsible for the patient should be communicated with to inform them of the situation and what can and cannot be done about it.

In all cases, if you are wrong, and if legal consultation is not necessary, admit it, and try to make restitution as quickly and effectively as possible. In all cases, respond quickly, show your concern, and let the complainant know what you are doing. Very often your real concern will serve to indicate your sincerity and, instead of having an enemy, you will have created a friend who understands that mistakes do happen and that your nursing home most certainly does everything in its power to avoid them and correct them.

XXVI

EMERGENCY PUBLIC RELATIONS

EVERY NURSING HOME should have certain administrative guidelines which are to be placed into effect in case of emergency. Such guidelines should be reviewed regularly, with responsible employees being drilled on what they are to do, how they are to do it, and when. Part and parcel of these rules and regulations should be information regarding press relations. The following advice is offered to help you formulate your own rules and regulations:

SPOKESMAN. Information should be given on who will act as spokesman for the nursing home. This means one person and one person only. All questions should be referred to this person. In cases where news media personnel are present, no employee should volunteer any information of any kind, nor should he respond to questions with any answer other than, "I'm sorry, but I just don't have the time now to answer the questions," or "I'm not able to answer that question. Ask Mr. . . ." To answer a question in any other way could mean a misstatement of fact, though completely unintended, which could harm the home's reputation when in fact the home was not at fault. Although lack of fault may be proved later, it may be the initial misstatement which gets the coverage, and which is remembered. Only one person should act as a spokesman because only one person is in a position to know all the facts.

ON THE SCENE. The spokesman should not answer any on the scene questions except to say that everything possible is being done to solve the current crisis and that there is no way of knowing cause at this time.

STATEMENT. Any statement given to the press should be in written form, prepared with the advice of legal counsel.

INTERVIEWS. No interview should be granted except in the office of the spokesman who would have all necessary facts and figures at his disposal. The spokesman should have prepared answers for obvious questions. Also, any interview should be recorded by tape recorder to assure that any stories developed therefrom, or that any question, are reported correctly, and not taken out of context. Say nothing "off the record."

—— PART II ——

PUBLICS AND RELATIONS

INTRODUCTION TO PART II

Part II contains information regarding specific programs to undertake to improve relations with various publics with which you must contend. The programs discussed are not intended to be the be-all and end-all. Rather, they are offered as possibilities, acceptable as is or with modification, or to serve as a stimulus to your own imagination. Most of the tools discussed in Part I are applicable to many of your publics, and it is suggested that you rely on the index to help coordinate information and facilitate your efforts.

XXVII

PATIENT RELATIONS

BECAUSE IMAGE PRIMARILY is a reflection of what actually exists, it stands to reason that how patients regard you and your facility depends primarily on the quality of overall care they receive. As with no other public, the method which you must use to create good relations with patients—establishment and maintenance of quality care—is a major determining factor of what many other publics will think of the nursing home. If everything is done to take all patient problems into consideration; if every effort is bent to help patients retrieve as much independence and self-respect as possible, it cannot help but be an important factor—if not the most important factor—in determining your home's image in the minds of patients' families, prospective patients and their families, volunteers, other health care professionals, community groups and even employees. Even in professional circles, real dedication to patients' well-being is recognized as a positive element which often can outweigh certain deficiencies.

Employee Attitudes

Because it is the employee public which comes into contact most frequently and most directly with patients, it is essential that all personnel receive instructions regarding correct attitudes toward patients. This requires more than just a mention in an employee handbook. It requires that all employees as a group, or as several groups in terms of shift personnel, must be informed and continually reminded of dos and don'ts. It also means that each new employee must be so instructed and that each employee who seemingly is not following instructions must be reinstructed and observed.

The basic message which must be transmitted is that each patient is an individual, adult human being and deserves to be treated as such. Complaints are not to be taken lightly or overlooked. Personal preferences must be observed. In essence, the nursing home is, for the patients, a home and a community in which they must live. Because patients' freedom of choice is limited, it is up to employees to help those requiring care receive the maximum possible positive benefit from their environment, and the least possible negative impact.

Employees must strive to treat patients much as they would like to be treated were they in the same circumstances, more or less a nursing home golden rule.

Specific ways and means of instructing employees, in addition to group talks and sensitivity sessions, include comments in an employee newsletter, memoranda, bulletins, pay envelope stuffers, and person-to-person communication. In other words, a general attitude first must be shaped thorough creation of a general understanding, with specifics given to cement attitudes and provide tools whereby each staff member can help make a meaningful contribution. If the general attitude is successfully established, then the specifics will be welcomed and the tools utilized.

Orientation

Whenever possible each new patient should be oriented to the facility in light of his own attitudes and interests. The orientation assignment, therefore, requires a degree of sensitivity and should be given only to a person capable of performing the task. Basic orientation could include a tour of those parts of the facility with which the patient will come into contact, such as his room, dining area, activities areas, therapy rooms, and so forth, as well as people such as roommates, nurse, nurse's aides, activities director and volunteers. More specifically, if the patient has had a life-long interest in gardening, the gardens should be one of the key spots on the tour, and those other patients interested in gardening should be introduced as soon as possible. In other words, the initial orientation tour should be designed to immediately give patients something to look forward to, and so offset the oft-prevalent fear of having nothing to look forward to.

Patient Recognition

An effort should be made on the part of all key staff members to know the full name of each patient, with the same effort being made by those employees who come into contact with patients most frequently. The name used to address a patient should be that name by which the patient prefers to be addressed. This means that no one in the facility should assume automatically that a patient named Mrs. Anne Smith prefers to be called Annie by one and all. Perhaps she may prefer her friends and certain employees to call her Annie or Anne, while preferring certain others to call her Mrs. Smith. This is information which you should attempt to learn either through contact with family or friends or just by asking "Mrs. Smith" herself.

Additional recognition can be fostered through programs mentioned elsewhere in this book, including a patient of the month program, spotlight features in the newsletter, and others. Likewise, it is part and parcel of an activities program to recognize the accomplishments of individuals, if only on a one-to-one congratulatory basis, and so positively reinforce any progress made.

Still another form of recognition centers on events in the patient's life, such as birthdays. Not only should families be encouraged to recognize them, but you should take the time to send a birthday card, as well as cards for occasions such as Valentine's Day, Easter, and other holidays of lay and religious origin. Bear in mind that such recognition on behalf of nursing home administration should be even-handed, given to all patients alike, so no favoritism is shown.

Communication

Communication with patients is essential because the nursing home is their home and community and they accordingly must be aware of what is happening. Forms of communication already have been discussed in detail elsewhere, but when it comes to patients certain specifics should be observed because their needs are unique. Written communications must be produced in a type size large enough to enable easy-reading by those whose eyesight is limited. Person-to-person communication must take into consideration an individual patient's hearing problems. For example, those who can hear only slightly must be spoken to so that the speaker is close to the better ear, while also facing the patient to enable lip reading. If such niceties are not observed, administration's attempt to communicate may result in frustration, which could be worse than no communication at all.

A most important element in the patient communications program is the bulletin board, often placed near a room frequently used, such as the dining room. The board should be positioned to allow easy viewing by those in wheelchairs. Items to be included on the bulletin board should be those relevent to patient activities, as well as photographs, menus, news clippings and similar material. The board should be kept current at all times, especially since many members of outside publics will be seeing it on tours of the facility.

Activities Program

Without exception, every nursing home should be encouraged to undertake an activities program for patients. In fact, an activities program becomes the major element of a patient relations program, for it is through an activities program that a patient is given challenge and so the opportunity to maintain what capabilities are left, and regain many of those impaired or thought lost. This book shall not even attempt to discuss activities programs, because it would fall far short of the mark. Fortunately, much literature on the subject currently is available and under development. Suffice it to say here that without an activities program; without a chance for meaningful-to-the-patient involvement, a nursing home becomes little more than a warehouse. All nursing homes, regardless of size or resources, must begin establishment of activities programs, regardless of how small or limited in scale, if they are to become institutions worthy of respect.

XXVIII

PATIENT FAMILY RELATIONS

FAMILIES OF PATIENTS comprise a very important public for several reasons. First, because of experience, their opinion of your nursing home is very credible. Second, on a day-to-day basis, their perception of the quality of care being received by the patient determines continued use of your facility. Third, through effective patient family relations, family members are more apt to become involved with the nursing home and its programs of patient care, and therefore can contribute to the emotional well-being of the family member as well as other patients.

Regular Communication
Regular communication with patient families (and friends, in some cases) should include materials such as general newsletter, press releases, clippings and related materials. Also, occasional photographs of patients may be sent (showing involvement in an activity of some sort) as well as periodic (monthly, bimonthly) progress reports which indicate what activities the patient has participated in, therapeutic progress, and so forth.

Another regular communication should be reminder notices of events such as birthdays, special holidays (Valentine's Day, Mother's Day, religious holidays, and others) sent out two weeks beforehand. The communication need only be a post card, stating, for example:

"Just a note to remind you that Mrs. Smith's birthday is January 18. I'm sure she would love to have a visit (10 AM to 7 PM), plus a card, call, or note.

Sincerely,
John Doe, Administrator

Families also should be sent brief but friendly invitations to appropriate functions, such as outings, banquets, and the like.

Visitation Reminders
Records should be kept to determine how frequently a patient

is visited by family members. If visits of those who live fairly close by are few and far between, a letter should be written, or a call made, to encourage visitation. If visits seem to cause a patient irritation or conflict, for any one of a variety of reasons, an effort should be made—with family members and patients—to determine why and to develop strategies to make visitation a positive experience.

Letter Writing

Family communications with patients via letters should be encouraged. In fact, an ideal situation would involve a schedule of letter writing whereby the patient would receive letters frequently, perhaps as many as one a day or four a week, from different family members. Through other patients or certain staff members you probably will be able to ascertain if a patient is receiving letters from those held most dear. If not, emphasize the importance of receipt of letters in the daily nursing home routine, and encourage frequent communications.

Dunning Notices

There may be occasion to send a family a notice regarding late payment. In this case and in other appropriate cases, it is suggested that the notice be personal, rather than a mass-produced card or form. A mass-produced form says, between the line: "So many people are late in payment that we've had these notices printed in quantity." Because of this fact, and because of the impersonality of the communication, such notices easily are ignored. It is therefore recommended that anyone late in paying receive a personal letter. Typical copy could be:

```
Dear Mr. Jones:
In reviewing our records, we note that payment
for the month of June has not as yet been
received. If for some reason you are unable to
make payment, please give us a call. We will
try our best to work with you to ensure that
Mrs. Jones continues to receive the care
required. If payment and this letter are
```

```
crossing in the mails, our thanks, and I am
sure Mrs. Jones looks forward to seeing you
soon.
                            Sincerely,
```

In cases of continued late payments, it is advised that several versions of the letter be readied to avoid continued sending of the exact same message. In cases where the first letter is ignored, a phone call would be appropriate.

XXIX

PROSPECTIVE PATIENT
FAMILY RELATIONS

T YPICALLY, THOSE WHO become most involved in the nursing home selection procedure are the sons and daughters of those who require nursing home care. Because of strong emotional involvement, it would be a relatively simple task to take advantage of such persons. In fact, some have, and in so doing have devastated not only their own reputations, but also have helped cast aspersions on the entire industry.

To establish an image of being a responsible, reliable, concerned, professional member of the health care profession, the administrator must strive to be exactly what he wants people to think of him as. This requires an understanding of the emotional stresses which the prospective patient family and the prospective patient are undergoing, and the complete willingness to be as honest and helpful as possible.

In this way, should your nursing home not be selected, at least you have made a friend.

Emotional State

Numerous tracts have been written on the emotional state of those involved in the selection of a nursing home and, to be of maximum assistance to the prospective patient family, you should read some of the literature. Bear in mind that observed behavior does not necessarily correlate with actual emotional state. It is only through understanding of some basic psychological phenomena that an individual can be of real help to those experiencing emotional stress. The following discussion is not at all intended to supplant the need for further reading on the subject, but is designed to indicate a few factors which must be considered to establish effective prospective family relations.

First of all, few families follow advice of experts and select a nursing home before placement becomes an immediate necessity. One probable cause for this is the mistaken belief that the nursing home represents finality; that placement in a nursing home virtually symbolizes that the patient involved will never leave alive. Hence, the longer the nursing home is avoided, the longer the reality of a loved one's serious illness is avoided. And when a nursing home must be found, the patient's family often suffers from very strong guilt feelings, a son or daughter eventually feeling that nursing home selection and placement is like signing a death warrant.

The guilt feelings can manifest themselves in several ways. One common result is hasty selection of a home based on other than most pertinent criteria, coupled with complete lack of involvement of the patient. In some cases, when a patient does accompany offspring on an inspection tour or preplacement interview, he, too, is treated like a block of wood, minimizing pain to offspring by denying strong emotional bonds.

Realizing the depth and strength of emotions involved, it is imperative that whoever deals with prospective patient families be sensitive to their needs and attempt to help make the selection process achieve its real purpose. This means that the exact needs of the patient be discussed; that determination of the home's ability to meet these needs be made, and that all discussion about related factors, including costs, be as open and honest as possible, tempered by knowledge of the family's emotional condition.

In cases where patients accompany the family, the patient must be involved in conversation to as great a degree as possible. After all, the patient is an adult human being and should be treated as such.

Other considerations are discussed below.

Selection Literature

A variety of materials are available from the government and various national associations regarding criteria to consider in selecting a nursing home. These should be reviewed by management to measure their conformity to the various positive aspects; help identify those factors which should be considered, to help determine what can be done to be of maximum assistance to prospective patient families. In addition, it is strongly suggested that a supply of these books be on hand for distribution to those involved in the selection process. (You also should consider having on hand various materials on Medicare, Medicaid and related programs.)

Hours—Staffing

Someone should be appointed with the responsibility for effective prospective patient family relations and should be on duty at least during visiting hours should visits be made without prior appointment, as some advise. It would be appropriate to conduct training and/or sensitivity sessions to ensure that personnel with prospective patient family relations responsibilities are capable of carrying them out in the correct manner. Should interviews with families be conducted by appointment only, fewer people will require training, but the home runs the risk of losing a potential patient or getting a relationship off to a bad start.

Establishing the Relationship

Assuming that a prospective patient family either appears on the door step or has an appointment, the relationship can begin with discussion in a private office. Interest and concern should be displayed at the outset, with the home's representative leading discussion. Once basic information on the prospective patient is ascertained, the family should be told whether or not the nursing home can provide needed services and, if so, they should be told of the home's various programs, credentials, and other general material. Following initial discussion, the family should be taken on a tour of the facility perhaps being given one of the selection guides published by HEW or ANHA. In pointing out room, equipment or services, care should be taken to relate them to the prospective patient and his requirements.

Following the tour of the facility, discussion should be continued in the office, beginning with answering any questions relating to nursing home care. In some cases, it even may be advisable to broaden the subject of common misunderstandings regarding nursing homes, explaining them honestly, and in detail.

Discussion regarding guilt feelings and associated emotional problems also may be worthwhile.

One subject which of course must be discussed is money. The best policy is to be completely frank, itemizing point by point each element of cost on a specified basis (per month, one time only, annual, and so forth) complete with options (private room vs. double, etc.) as well as full explanations of what third party payments can be expected.

Nearing the end of the discussion, prospective patient families could be provided with various written materials for study or reference at home, including selection guides (if not previously provided), brochure, patient family guide (including information on visiting hours), as well as a sheet specifying costs and related information.

In cases where the initial visit is made without the prospective patient, and depending on other circumstances, it may be appropriate to suggest another visit, including the prospective patient.

Follow-Up

Following a visit, and again depending on circumstances, some continued contact is advised at least in the form of a letter stating that it was "a pleasure meeting with you" and that "if there is any way in which we can be of service, please do not hesitate to ask."

XXX

EMPLOYEE RELATIONS

TOO OFTEN WE hear the story of the nursing home administrator whose employees have unionized. He is completely in the dark as to why his employees would want the union approach. Often he says, "I can't understand it. My door is always open. They know that." But do they really? In many instances, while the administrator may be very open-hearted and even-handed toward employees, he has never or has only rarely communicated his generous attitude. The administrator has taken it for granted, and employees have never recognized it for a fact.

In this light, therefore, it readily can be seen that management must do everything in its power to let employees know exactly where they stand, what the management expects from them and what they can expect from management. Further, programs must be developed to express through action management's concern for the well-being of employees. The development of an image of understanding and concern through development of programs symbolizing such sentiment is purely a public relations function, in this case the target public being employees.

If such programs can be established, they also will help overcome the very serious problems of employee turnover. Many programs which evidence management's concern also create a bond of affinity between the employee and the nursing home, so that many enjoyable, worthwhile benefits would be lost the moment employment is terminated. Use of the following suggested programs, combined with use of many of the tools discussed in Part I, will lead to greatly improved employee relations and development of employees who are happy to be associated with you and to act as your ambassadors of good will in the community.

Policy Handbook

Too often management overlooks the importance of its actions as they affect the life of an employee. In fact, you are one of the most important elements of an employee's life: The satisfaction to be derived from the job you give him determines the satisfaction he derives from most of his life; what you pay determines how he lives; the promise you can provide for his future helps determine the way in which he conducts himself each day, striving to turn promise into reality.

While many subjects will be covered during orientation, others will not be and some which are explained will fall victim to the mysterious wiles of the memory. Too often important questions, such as "What do you have to do around here to get a raise?" are answered by rumor. Therefore, it is most strongly suggested that one of the best investments that you possibly could make in terms of employee relations is development of an employee policy handbook which lets an employee know exactly where he stands and which answers as many questions as possible about his job, his working environment, and what he must do to advance himself and make his own life better. Further, development of an employee handbook will allow management to think through its own policies which heretofore may have been vague and, in so doing, develop uniform policies which will not be subject to unequal application and an aura of favoritism which can, whether it actually exists or not, undermine employee confidence in management.

CONTENTS. Below are listed some of the items which should be included in a policy handbook:

Introduction, probably the most critical element of the employee policy handbook. Because most of the policy handbook will be worded very tersely, spelling out rules and regulations, dos and don'ts, the introduction can serve to soften all that follows and illustrate management's genuine concern for the welfare of all employees. A typical introduction can be worded as follows:

"This policy handbook has been created to provide you with some basic information regarding your employment at XYZ Nursing Home. Because much of what follows explains rules and regulations, it is written in what might seem to be a very abrupt, unfriendly manner. Unfortunately, there is no other way to write rules and regulations if they are to be spelled out clearly and exactly and be applied to all employees in a fair manner. Please do not feel that the management of XYZ Nursing Home is unfriendly or unconcerned about you. We feel that each employee is an individual, a human being like everyone else who walks on this planet. If you have problems with which you feel we can help; if you have questions which this policy handbook does not answer, or for whatever appropriate reason, the door is always open. Please come and see me and talk. Don't accept rumor or hearsay or gossip. We will try to do our best to answer your questions; to help when we can, and to make our relationship mutually rewarding and satisfying.

The nursing home is a fit subject for a second introduction to the policy handbook, wherein mention should be made of the nursing home itself and its reason for existence. Discussion should begin with a history of the home, detailing when it was built, expansion which has taken place over the years, etc. The next item to discuss should be the purpose of the nursing home, namely to provide patients not only with care for the problems which necessitate their use of a nursing home, but also to provide them with a home and a community, unlike all other health care facilities. Employees should be reminded that all patients are individuals themselves, worthy of the respect to which all individuals are entitled. At your discretion, you also may wish to make note of the type home involved, i.e., proprietary or nonproprietary. When discussing a proprietary home, mention should be made of the fact that profits achieved in operation are returned to those who invested their funds enabling establishment of the nursing home in the first place. Nonproprietary homes should stress the fact that while the home is not operated for a profit, it still must observe the same fiscal responsibility any business must if it is to ensure its continued ability to provide care to those who need it.

Departmental information should include detailing how the nursing home is divided into departments and what responsibilities are carried out in each. Care should be taken to stress that each department is crucial to the overall operation of the nursing home. For example, while it ostensibly is the responsibility of the housekeeping department to keep the nursing home clean, it should be mentioned that its responsibilities are most important due to the fact that it is responsible for reducing accidents in the nursing home and minimizing germs and the possibilities of infection, to which nursing home patients are particularly susceptible.

As an Employee is a section of the handbook which can come just prior to the rules and regulations. Typical wording for such a section is as follows:

As an employee of XYZ Nursing Home, you represent the nursing home. When speaking on the telephone; when talking with visitors or others who enter our home, even when not on the premises, you represent our nursing home. What you say and do represents our nursing home. In fact, to a very real degree you are entrusted with our reputation. This is not to imply that you must be a model of virtue at all times when in our employ. But we do ask that you conduct yourself in a manner which reflects well not only on yourself, but on your place of employment. Just as an example, you no doubt have been treated rudely by an employee of some establishment and, as a result, you probably make it a point not to use their services or buy their products. The facts of the matter are that the establishment probably is good, but the actions of just one person, acting foolishly or without thinking of his or her responsibility to the place of employment, resulted in your avoiding everything having to do with that place. So, we ask you to bear in mind that, as our employee, you are a member of our family, and what you do or say can have a lot to do with what other people think of you, your fellow employees, and everything concerned with XYZ Nursing Home.

Rules and Regulations should be itemized, including:

1. *Work Day and Week* Discussion should center on how many hours in the work day and week, when employees are expected to report, and so forth. If there are differences from one department to another, or from shift to shift, these should be spelled out clearly, perhaps by explaining the work week on a department by department basis.

2. *Overtime* Discussion of this subject probably is best carried out by differentiating between salaried and nonsalaried employees. Mention should be made of the fact that as much advance notice as possible will be given and, when overtime is required, nonsalaried workers will receive appropriate compensation, detailing exactly what compensation that is, such as time and one-half. Salaried employees usually are not given overtime, and this or whatever basis is used, also should be mentioned.

3. *Sick Leave* Discussion of sick leave information should include:

a) When sick leave first is attainable, for example, after the first six months;

b) how many days per year, per six months, or during whatever time division is established;

c) whether sick leave can be accumulated from year-to-year, just during two years, or what have you, and;

d) how sick leave not used is reimbursed, or otherwise compensated.

4. *Pregnancy Leave* Your home should have a policy regarding

pregnancy, including how long leave is granted, whether or not the position is protected, and so on.

5. *Vacations* Cover who is entitled to vacations; how much time is granted for vacation after varying lengths of service; how vacation time can be accumulated; how vacation time can be reimbursed if not used; how much notice must be given in establishing time for vacations.

6. *Holidays* Discuss and list what days in the year are given as holidays; how it is determined who will work during holidays, special compensation for those who do, and so forth.

7. *Insurance Program* Include what the nursing home offers in terms of health and life insurance, pension and related programs, and how and when employees are eligible.

8. *Educational Programs* Discuss whether or not time off with or without pay is given for attending special educational programs, such as seminars, workshops and actual courses; how the nursing home attempts to recognize educational advancement; if educational loans, grants, partial tuitions are available, and related items.

9. *In-house Career Development* Include what the nursing home does by way of providing lateral mobility, so a person can move from a position in one department to a position in another, thereby increasing his overall knowledge and abilities.

10. *Promotions* Detail what criteria are used in promoting a person; whether or not the attempt first is made to promote from in-house staff, and so forth.

11. *Job Descriptions* Prepared individually for each job, each job description should detail exactly what a person's responsibilities are, to whom he reports, etc. (See Chapter XXXII.)

12. *Safety* Discussion of various fire and accident safety rules and regulations (with possible separate inserts for each department) ; handling and use of drugs, and related concerns.

In addition, you may want to include in the handbook more specific information on relationships with patients, when to take initiatives and when not to; safety and smoking rules and regulations; relationships with families of patients; and related material which are of concerns.

WRITING STYLE. As indicated above, the writing style for the most of the book, except for the introductory material, should be terse and easily understood. It can even be outlined if necessary. The thing is to make everything completely understandable so as to answer as many questions as possible.

FORMAT. The simplest format for such a book is a typewritten page, printed inexpensively and bound in an inexpensive paper binder.

This allows for easy page changes or insertion of new material. Also, it is inexpensive enough to allow you to give a handbook to each employee. It is not at all necessary to make an elaborate production out of the policy handbook. The important thing is to give a clean, new copy to each employee.

Communications

It is imperative that an effective communications program be established in the nursing home to allow for management-to-employee, employee-to-management and employee-to-employee communication. In addition to the newsletter, already discussed, here follow some typical programs worthy of consideration.

EMPLOYEE COUNCIL. One of the most effective selling points which a union can offer is its promise that employees, through unionization, will have a much larger voice in the way the facility is managed. Nor is this an unreasonable goal. Because the manner in which a facility is managed is so crucial to the satisfaction which employees derive from their work, they should have a say.

An excellent vehicle which management can utilize to give employees a voice, without resorting to unionization, is the employee council, representing the interests of employees through their selection of a representative or two from each department. The council could be consulted on matters such as development of an employee-of-the-month program, suggestion programs, bulletin board programs, and so forth. Further, it can be consulted on more substantive issues, including administrative rules and regulations. The comments of an employee council can be very worthwhile if a program which you otherwise would have begun would have resulted in bitterness and thinning of the ranks. Establishment of such an organization must be undertaken with the realization that any recommendation of the council can be ignored by management if it so wishes, but that most recommendations, particularly those which do not relate to administrative rules and regulations, will be followed. Naturally, any recommendation which may be overruled should be discussed fully before it is overruled, and any overruling or veto should be accompanied by a thorough explanation.

While the program has many benefits, there are some potential pitfalls which must be considered. First, while the program demonstrates management's willingness to have employee involvement in decisions concerning employee programs, it will backfire seriously if those items allowed for consideration are inconsequential, or if council recommendations or decisions are continually overruled. Second, if the program is begun, but is dropped because of continual management-employee conflict, it could in fact lead to unionization and reestablishment of the council concept in terms of a union. Therefore, it is advised that any such program be undertaken with care, and that complete guidelines be established regarding mutual responsibilities. Through careful implementation of this concept you will be able to demonstrate your sincere desire for employee job satisfaction, and in so doing solve many work-related problems before they become problems, and before they lead to unionization.

GENERAL MEETINGS. In cases where the number of employees is small enough, or where an employee council does not exist, it makes sense to hold general meetings of all employees to discuss matters of mutual concern. Such matters could include placement of new snack machines; development of new programs, such as institution of a volunteer program, and so forth. You can use these meetings to obtain employee involvement in the operation of the home, as well as to answer any questions which may arise, or note any suggestions. The meetings should be kept short, and held at reasonably convenient times. Naturally, such meetings demonstrate concern for employees, and respect for their good will and opinions.

CLOUDS ON THE HORIZON MEETINGS. It is suggested that once a month management hold a meeting with department heads, whether or not they are the ones who make up an employee council. The type meeting is called "Clouds on the Horizon" and is used primarily to discuss emerging situations within each department, what management has in mind for the future, and related items. In other words, it is a general planning unit, utilized to ensure continued smooth running of operations. Further, it involves key employees with management, making them feel all the more part of the home.

NEWS IN GENERAL. Employees should be the first to know about any major new developments within the nursing home. If, for example, they first hear about a new assistant administrator by reading about it in the newspaper, they cannot help but feel as if they had been overlooked by management and simply taken for granted. For this reason they should be kept informed of what is happening. This can be done in several ways: in meetings, through bulletins posted on the bulletin board, or through a newsletter. Be sure to use that vehicle which allows for the speediest delivery of news. For example, if the decision to hire an assistant administrator or to begin a volunteer program has been made; and assuming that a newsletter is not due out for two weeks, and a general meeting is not scheduled for a week, then a bulletin should be posted and the news announced. By treating employees in this manner they will feel, as they should, that they are somewhat special, and worthy of being given the "inside information" first.

BULLETIN BOARD. An employees-only bulletin board most obviously provides opportunity for management-to-employee and employee-to-employee communication. More subtly, it helps depict management as being concerned for employees by providing a separate communications vehicle and one which is semi-private vis-a-vis placement in an area remote from general view.

From the management point of view, an employees-only bulletin board is ideal for display of memoranda concerning scheduling, policy changes, new employees, safety and care tips, and related materials. From the employee point of view, it provides a vehicle for announcement of employee activities, posting items for sale, workshops and seminars for given occupations, and whatever other items employees deem appropriate.

To make a bulletin board program effective, several considerations must be borne in mind:

Location is essential An employees–only bulletin board must be placed in an area used mostly by employees only, such as an employees' lounge or dressing area.

Physical criteria are important also, in that the board must be large enough to provide adequate space for the bulletins to be posted. If the board continually is crowded, a larger one should be obtained.

Policy covering use must be established. For example, it must be determined whether the board will be placed behind locked glass or will be open for anyone's use at any time. The former method limits access but ensures control, bulletins being placed only through the consent of whomever is in charge, while the latter allows for free access, as well as the possibility that some bulletins may be removed before they should be.

Control of the bulletin board should be vested in one or several employees, on a permanent or rotating basis. If possible, the person in charge should be elected by employees, who also, with management's approval, should be allowed to establish most operating policies. Whoever is in charge of the program must be responsible for seeing to it that outdated bulletins are removed, and that those posted are appropriate. By having a control apparatus, the bulletin board program will have far more meaning and will be recognized as a viable means of communication.

SUGGESTION BOX PROGRAM. A suggestion box program provides for meaningful employee-to-management communication. Carried out correctly, the program: demonstrates to employees your belief in their having something worthwhile to say; shows your willingness to reward interest and valuable ideas and, not at all to be overlooked, provides potential for receiving effective, valuable suggestions.

The following guidelines should be considered in establishing a suggestion box program:

Placement of the suggestion box should be made in a location which permits patients as well as employees to make suggestions, or in a place similar to the employees' bulletin board. If it is to be primarily an employee program, the latter positioning is preferred, perhaps with rules governing the program placed permanently on the bulletin board. *Suggestion box* itself should be locked. If rules governing its use will appear on the box, they can be placed there utilizing decoupage techniques.

Rules concerning the program should include one which states that all suggestions, to be considered, must be signed and that unsigned suggestions will be discarded.

Policy should be established ensuring that all signed suggestions will be considered and replied to, preferably in letter sent to the employee's home. Naturally, should you see the employee prior to his receipt of the letter, you can comment on his submission in person, but be certain to send the letter. The letter can indicate why the suggestion won't work, or what has to be done to make it work. The letter indicates the suggestion was considered and that the thoughtfulness on the employee's part in making the suggestion is responded to in kind management.

Rewards for good suggestions should be commensurate with the value of the suggestion itself. It probably is best not to establish a standard suggestion–of–the–month award program simply because suggestions received in three consecutive months may be all but useless while in the fourth month there may be several good ones. Awards should be made when appropriate, therefore, and in all cases when good, usable suggestions are received. Also, you may wish to consider a "suggestion of the year" award, an extra bonus for the best suggestion received during the year.

Do not overlook the suggestion box program. It is an excellent low-cost tool for development of communications and effective employee relations. Moreover, the value of suggestions received may far exceed any cost expended on behalf of the program.

METHODS OF PRAISE AND SCOLDING. There will be occasions when certain employees, individually or as a group, will perform above and beyond the call of duty, as in certain emergency situations, or during an open house or other special functions, and so forth.

Whenever this occurs, management should make it a point to offer praise. The first and most obvious vehicle is to seek out each person and compliment him in person. The second step should entail a personal letter written to the employee at his home. This should not be a form letter which, in fact, can do more harm than good, indicating only massproduced, and therefore artificial thanks. Each letter of thanks should be individually typed or, if a large quantity is involved, typed by a multiple typewriter, a service available in-house if you have an IBM MT/ST, or available through a variety of outside services, often from a printer. In addition, each letter of thanks should be individually hand signed, if not by the administrator, then for him.

In addition to this, should there be occasion for a general meeting of employees, you should take the time to make note of the fact that certain of them did excellent work and deserve praise.

On the other hand, there will be occasions when certain employees deserve scolding. First of all, any such scolding should be made in private, never in public. By scolding in public you humiliate the employee and embarrass others who may hear. You come off all the worse, being regarded by those who hear you as thoughtless. Nor should a scolding be delivered in the form of a scolding. It should take the form of appropriate interpersonal communication. For some persons, it may be wiser to state, "I was very disappointed in your actions," rather than, "You really screwed it up yesterday." In other words, put yourself in the employee's shoes and deliver your message in a manner which will produce the best corrective actions and increased motivation, while avoiding creation of hostility and continued counterproductive behavior which will have to result in dismissal.

As a general rule, remember: Praise in public; scold in private.

EMPLOYEE COMPLAINTS. The employee handbook should cover the ways and means by which an employee can register dissatisfaction. However, there are cases when either the employee will not bring a complaint to the attention of the person who should hear it, or will continue to complain even after he has made his gripe known. In either case, the information about the employee's complaining should be obtainable through a clouds on the horizon type meeting or from other sources. In all cases the employee should be called into the office. If he has an honest gripe and you have not done everything possible to resolve it, do your best to resolve it as soon as possible. But if the complaint cannot be resolved, or if everything possible has been done, and the employee still complains, he should be told to either stop his complaining or look for work elsewhere (providing unions are not involved). A complainer can infect an entire staff and create untold problems. When this happens, it usually is necessary to inform several persons of why a person was dismissed, to ensure that the word gets around quickly that everything possible was done. In all cases, act as quickly as possible, either to resolve the complaint, or remove a chronic complainer.

Recognition Programs

There are a variety of recognition programs available to the nursing home, each designed to further the concept that an employee is an individual and should be treated as such. After all, those employees who feel that they only are another cog in the wheel cannot be expected to feel any ties with the nursing home, and will promptly leave when another job beckons. Nor can they be blamed for such action. Conversely, when an employee feels that he is known as a person; that his work is important and is regarded as such by others, then he has the beginning of a tie which will make him think twice before looking for work elsewhere.

EMPLOYEE IDENTIFICATION. It has been said that nothing is so sweet to a person's ear as the sound of his own name. In terms of employee relations there are a variety of simple recognition programs worthy of note.

Memory improvement can result in knowing employees by name or nickname, a most valuable attribute. In fact, it's easy to feel no real bond to an establishment when those who run it don't even know who you are. However, when the administrator sees you in the hall and says, "Hello, John. How are you feeling today?" it cannot help but make the person so addressed feel comfortable and secure in the knowledge that he is recognized as an individual. Therefore, it is suggested that you make an effort to know employees on sight, and take every advantage to treat them in a cordial, friendly manner, be it in the nursing home or elsewhere. If the task requires some instruction in memory improvement, as available through books and numerous short courses, it is strongly advised that you take it. It will stand you in excellent stead in many instances far beyond the value to be received in employee relations alone.

Name badges should be supplied to each employee. There are some very inexpensive badge making systems available, consisting of no more than blank tags on which one places a plastic tape/label bearing the employee's name. This enables one to know whom they are seeing or talking with, and lets employees know that you want them to be known as persons with names.

Business cards should be supplied to at least each department head, the card bearing the name of the nursing home and the name and title of the person involved. Even if used only on occasion, a business card is an ego-building device which has value only so long as the employee remains an employee.

Staff directory should be placed conspicuously near the reception area of the nursing home indicating each department, followed by the name of the person heading the department. It is flattering to see one's own name displayed, and the flattery exists only so long as the relationship with the nursing home exists.

In essence, an employee identification program amounts to no more than paying tribute to the fact that each employee is a person, and deserves recognition of that fact.

OF-THE-MONTH-PROGRAMS. There are a variety of employee recognition programs which can be inaugurated in the nursing home to provide individuals with public acknowledgement of their abilities. Typical of these programs are employee-of-the-month, nurse-of-the-year, and so forth. Such programs, when conducted correctly, can increase general employee morale. If handled incorrectly, or put together too hastily, however, they can backfire and create hostility where none previously existed.

In developing the policies and other concerns of a recognition program, it is suggested that management work with some type of employees council, as discussed previously. Some of the policy matters which must be settled include:

Who will be recognized? Obviously, a recognition program works best when all employees are eligible. While a nurse-of-the-month program would be effective for nursing staff, it would instantly make other employees feel like second class citizens. Such a program, therefore, would have to be balanced by laundry-worker-of-the-month, cook-of-the-month, etc., which would become too unwieldy. In most homes, therefore, it is suggested that the program be open for all employees.

Criteria must be established to ensure an appropriate basis of award, such as least amount of sick leave, or getting along well with fellow employees. But if such criteria are established, they should be established in conjunction with an employee council, allowing for their input on what makes an outstanding employee, and must be well-known among all employees. Even the best run such program can create some bitterness, however, particularly among those very good employees who do not receive recognition. Therefore, it may be best to establish an employee-of-the-month award based on a random sampling, from department to department each month on a rotating basis. While this dilutes somewhat an incentive to work harder to become employee-of-the-month, when such an award is based on merit, it also eliminates the possibility of antagonizing those who did try harder but were not rewarded. In larger homes, the award could be made on a weekly basis, or perhaps two employees could be chosen each month.

Form of recognition chosen is very important. There are a variety of ways in which an employee-of-the-month could be recognized regardless of what criteria are used in selection. Some of these recognition procedures include the following, usable individually or in combination:

  1. *In-House publicity,* including posting of photograph and

biographical information on both employee and patient bulletin boards and, if an in-house newsletter exists, in such a newsletter as a spotlight feature.

2. *Outside publicity,* including mailing of a press release and photograph to local newspapers.

3. *Awards ceremonies,* such as at a special one evening per month employees' dinner, featuring the presentation of an appropriate award. (See below.)

Also, assuming a recognition program based on a random sampling of various department personnel, it would be acceptable to have one or two year-end awards, perhaps two employee-of-the-year awards, one chosen by management only, the other chosen by patients only, each establishing their own criteria. Presentation could take palce at a function such as a Christmas party, complete with attendant awards presentation, publicity, etc.

EMPLOYEE AWARDS. Too often the selection of an award is given little or no consideration. Ideally, in selecting an award, you should attempt to choose something which, by its nature, is permanent and will continue to remind the employee of his relationship with your nursing home. As an example, if an employee's award is in the form of money, it is quickly spent and soon forgotten. The same is true of awards of vacations, savings bonds, banquets, and so forth. In other words, they become intangible and forgotten. Therefore, it strongly is recommended that the award, or at least part of the award, be something permanent and tangible, such as a plaque, or at least something which will last a long time, such as luggage. For example, an award of a savings bond and a plaque means that while the savings bond may disappear from view, the plaque will not and will have utmost meaning as long as the employee maintains his relationship with the nursing home. Therefore, it is suggested that at least part of any award take the form of something tangible and permanent, which the employee continually has before him, reminding him that he is appreciated by those for whom he works.

LONGEVITY AWARD. A special type award worthy of mention is that given for longevity of employment. Typical of this type award is the service pin, to be worn on a uniform. Usually a simple gold bar on which is impressed "5 YEARS", "10 YEARS", or whatever time period is appropriate. Presentation of such pins could be accompanied by a less tangible award, and perhaps special year-end presentation ceremonies, especially for those with ten or more years' service.

Group Volunteer Activities

Due to employees' affiliations with a variety of different organizations, there exists the possibility that the home and its employees, and possibly patients, too, can become involved in a variety of volunteer programs, working together as a unit. A group of employees may develop special interests in helping handicapped children or other groups, and they should be given leeway to interest other employees through use of the newsletter, bulletin board and similar communications tools. Likewise, you may consider allowing use of some of the home's facilities or grounds, thereby showing the home's interest in employees' concerns. Similarly, you may wish to encourage an in-house United Fund or United Way drive which often brings employees together as units, as well as creating news of the home.

Educational Policies and Programs

If at all possible, your nursing home should make an attempt to develop some overall policies in regard to education and employees, to allow for and encourage their development within the industry. Some typical programs worthy of consideration are discussed below.

LATERAL DEVELOPMENT. In larger homes it is a relatively simple matter to develop programs of lateral development, allowing an employee to shift from one department to another without loss of pay. In this manner he is enabled to broaden his background and so, hopefully, advance vertically.

VERTICAL DEVELOPMENT. Guidelines should be established on promotional policies and should be included in the employee policy handbook. Every effort should be made to fill positions with personnel already on staff. However, you should be very much aware of the "Peter Principle" which states, in essence, that many people are eventually advanced to a position of incompetence. In other words, if John Doe does excellently at Job A, he is promoted to Job B, where he also does well. Finally, he is promoted Job C, which really is not his "dish of tea" and, as a result, he stays there, continually doing a mediocre job in a task he really doesn't like. It is for this reason that lateral mobility is needed, so persons who have reached a "level of incompetence" can be put to work elsewhere, where they can once again start turning out excellent work, and continue to advance vertically.

EDUCATION LEAVE. Policy must be developed which takes educational leave into consideration, including workshops, seminars, two-week courses, night courses, even year-long college level courses. In the case of long-term leaves, such as for a semester at college, every attempt must be made to guarantee that the student will have, when he returns, a job which will recognize his increased education and abilities.

SCHOLARSHIPS, GRANTS. Policy must be developed regarding payment for educational courses. Will the home grant leave with pay for day-long courses? week-long courses? Will tuition be paid by the nursing home for courses which will improve the employee's work skills? Will it be paid for in part? Will a low-cost loan be given? Will dues to associations be paid when membership provides job enrichment or improved skills?

ADVANCEMENT. Also important, if the nursing home encourages employees to further their job related educational, how will the furtherance of this education be met? Especially in cases where costs for the additional training are not reimbursed by the nursing home, some attempt should be made to meet educational advancement and increased capabilities with increased pay, responsibilities, or both.

It should be borne in mind that simply being interested in an employee's continued education is not enough. The proof of the home's intentions and interests is in the extent of its willingness to meet an employee's initiatives with initiatives of its own, through payment for time not on the job, payment for attending a course, raises, and other actions.

EMPLOYEE LIBRARY. As an adjunct to educational policies, you may wish to consider creation of an employee library which consists of pertinent books available on a variety of subjects germane to the various jobs required in your nursing home, as well as related magazines. A 3 x 5 card index system can be used, as well as a simple withdrawal mechanism that allows a person to know who has a book in which he may be interested. The library could be run by employees themselves, with costs underwritten by the home.

Fringe Benefits

Fringe benefits seldom are appreciated by employees, often because management does not do enough to emphasize them, or to develop very obvious ones. Here follow suggestions to improve fringe benefits and to make employees more aware of them.

COST SAVINGS PROGRAMS. If your nursing home has enough employees, there are several programs available which will provide them with cost savings. An example of such programs is United Buying Service, or similar buying services which may be in operation in your area. These organizations contract with various distributors, particularly car dealers, to purchase and indeterminate number of items at a percentage above wholesale, splitting the profit when members of the service present a purchase order and buy. There usually is no cost to join, and the cost savings can be significant. For example, United Buying Service makes most American cars available to members at $100 above wholesale. Similar programs should be investigated, including a credit union; the possibility of buying uniforms in quantity, thereby reducing the price; having personnel from your facility's accountant's office doing income tax returns for employees at reduced rates, and so on. For the most part such programs cost your nursing home little or nothing, but they can become a very important benefit of working for the home, one which continues only as long as employment continues.

EMPLOYEE TIPS PROGRAM. Not a day goes by when the nursing home administrator does not read some periodical, or hear of an incident which results in some sort of tip or cautionary advice. Around income tax time, for example, there probably are many tips that are read in various newspapers or which can be supplied by your nursing home's accountant. Many of these can be geared for employees, advising them, for example, about certain deductions for uniforms, cars when used to transport patients, and related matters. Similarly, we hear tips about the dangers of mixing radial and nonradial tires; tips on how to save on heating bills, on ad infinitem. The wise administrator will save these tips and perhaps put them into the form of memoranda or pay envelope stuffers passing on usable advice to employees. The cost of running such a program is practically nothing, but the good will established can be priceless.

LETTING THE EMPLOYEE KNOW. A major complaint for many employers is the fact that an employee seldom realizes that what he makes, and what management actually pays out on his behalf, usually are two entirely different figures, fringe benefits and Social Security often costing one-quarter to one-third more than actual pay. An excellent vehicle through which to inform and remind employees of this additional expense including vacations, sick leave, holidays, insurance, and so on, is to prepare a special form for distribution with a W-2 form at year's end, showing exactly how much the employee has received. He often will be pleased and surprised to learn that he is earning far more than what he may have thought he was earning. In addition, you may wish to include a typical example in your employee handbook.

Extracurricular Activities

Another program devised to develop the employee's relationship with the nursing home involves development of social, athletic and other activities whose enjoyment becomes unattainable the moment the relationship with the nursing home ceases.

Typical social functions include holiday parties for employees and their families, patients and their families, or just employees only (with special consideration given to those who work late shifts) ; picnics; monthly birthday parties for employees only or employees and patients, and similar social events.

Sports activities, an excellent vehicle for establishing group identity, can be centered for both on-the-grounds and off-grounds events. On-the-grounds events could include ping-pong, shuffleboard, pool or bumper pool, badminton, volleyball, touch football, and similar activities which space and facilities permit. The development of tournaments also can serve to heighten interest. Off-grounds events would consist of bowling, softball, golf and related activities.

Also to be considered are employee contests, including word games (place a word on the bulletin board and the employee deriving the most words from its letters gets a prize) ; guessing games (how many beans in the jar) , bridge tournaments or other card tournaments, and so on.

Obviously, the more such programs, the more enjoyment the employee can derive from being employed by your nursing home. By the same token, more activities mean more cost. For this reason it is suggested that a thorough analysis be made of all prospective activities, evaluating each in terms of value toward an overall program of employee retention. Those which are deemed most important could be underwritten entirely by the home. Those which are deemed of less value could be underwritten partly by the home. Those which have a low level of value could be endorsed by the home, but contributed to only in the form of providing space, or ping pong balls, or other minimally expensive or cost-free contributions.

While direct control of most of these activities should be left to employees selected by their peers, management should maintain involvement to as great an extent as possible, to illustrate enthusiasm and a willingness to support such activities and, in some cases, to participate in them.

XXXI

NEW EMPLOYEE RELATIONS

THE NEW EMPLOYEE must be treated in a distinct manner to ensure that he begins his relationship with the nursing home "on the right foot." If every effort is made in this regard, then a firm foundation for the future will be established.

Training

Much of the relationship with a new employee often involves training, a subject beyond the scope and purpose of this book. Suffice it to say that the employee must be trained sufficiently to enable him to perform his tasks correctly, for his sake as well as your own. After all, an employee who cannot perform well is a frustrated individual, plus his value to management is slight. It is imperative, therefore, to determine the effect of training, which, of course, means a monitoring process, as well as a continuing program of encouragement based on the rules of interpersonal communication. Do not expect an employee to perform well at a function in which he has not been trained, or in which your specific requirements have not been related.

Orientation

Another key element of new employee relations is orientation, which, if procedures in the following chapter are followed, should be a relatively easy task. Briefly, new employee orientation involves a second tour of the facility, with emphasis on the new employee's department and his co-workers there, and information which illustrates how the employee's job is an integral element to the smooth operation of the entire facility. For example, a laundry worker must be told that clean linens are essential to patient well-being; what could happen if the job is performed poorly, and the chain reaction of problems which could set in.

Naturally, if the new employee does not already possess a copy of the employee handbook, including a job description, he should be given one, along with any other pertinent material. Also, the new employee should be introduced to as many other employees as possible (a task which is perhaps best handled by a long-time employee in the same department), and news of the hiring could be made public through the bulletin board, newsletter, and other means, including a news release for key personnel. You may even wish to consider giving a new employee a special color or type badge to wear, for the first week or so, so fellow employees immediately will recognize him as a new employee and greet him accordingly. (You may wish to include suggestions on this subject as a special insert in the employee handbook, as an occasional subject for comment in an employee newsletter insert, or as a subject for discussion in meetings.)

Also, it should be the job of the administrator and the respective department head, and other key personnel, to drop in on the new employee during his first few weeks of employment to make sure that he knows what he is doing, and that he is happy with his work. In such a manner one lays the foundation for a solid relationship.

XXXII

PROSPECTIVE AND FORMER EMPLOYEE RELATIONS

A WORD OR TWO must be given to discussion of relations with prospective and former employees who form two distinct publics capable of relating to others their impressions of you and your facility.

Prospective Employees and the Hiring Process

Prospective employees are those who enter the nursing home in response to advertising. Proper hiring techniques are essential because it is imperative that the person hired be suited for the work involved. If not, he will become disgruntled, or will simply be unable to perform assigned tasks. One way or another he will eventually leave, or will continue to do subpar work. Given the ever rising costs of hiring, orienting, training, terminating, and associated functions, it is imperative that some thought and consideration be given to hiring policies. While much information on this subject is available from other sources, at least some food for thought is contained below.

JOB DESCRIPTIONS. Writing the job description is a necessary and crucial task. You may think you know what the job entails, but may not be correct. To hire a person based on only an educated guess of what really will be required of him is to jeopardize an investment of time and money, and risk irritating what is obviously a prospective ambassador of good will. In preparing a job description—and one should be prepared for each job category in the facility—it is suggested that you write down exactly what you believe the job entails, then have several others do the same, including the head of the department in which the vacancy exists, and perhaps the immediate superior or co-workers. Compare the several job descriptions and note any discrepencies. Meet with those who have written the descriptions to discuss the issue and to determine precisely what is and is not required. Once this is determined it is a relatively simple matter to proceed to general attributes which the person filling the position must possess.

PERSONAL CHARACTERISTICS CHECKLIST. Once the job description is complete, it is advised that you meet with those several people who will be working most closely with the new worker to determine what other-than-job-related characteristics may be important. For example, given the character of a vital member of staff who would be working with the new worker, it may be essential that the new staffer be capable of maintaining a cheerful attitude. In other words, in selecting an employee, try to avoid co-worker conflicts which may appear to be inevitable. Naturally, the checklist of desired or undesirable attributes is kept confidential.

REQUIREMENTS/QUANTITY LIST. A requirements/quantity list indicates which abilities and/or characteristics are most important, which second most, etc. For example, if the person, to do the job, must have talents A, B, C, D, and E, the quality checklist would indicate the relative importance of each. You can use a 1 to 10 scale, so that quality A, most important, would rate a 10, with quality B a 3, quality C a 5, and so forth. During or after the interview rank the prospective employee's characteristics in terms of qualities possessed using the same scale. By using this method you may find, for example, that an applicant may possess all five qualities required, but they may be in definitely unfavorable proportions. A secretary who can take dictation and be able to type may be what you are looking for, but if you hire a person who cannot take dictation too well but can type very quickly, when in fact dictation is the key element, you have made a costly mistake. The requirements/quantity list can help minimize the chance of error.

EMPLOYMENT FORMS. All forms should be carefully scrutinized from the point of view of requirements of the Equal Employment Opportunity Commission and whatever state laws may exist. Certain questions which you may think are harmless could in fact be deemed discriminatory and make you and your nursing home liable to legal action. Therefore, we advise consulting with your state and national nursing home association, or directly with the EEOC.

TOUR. A tour of the facility is advised for all prospective employees, not dissimilar from the one which should be given as part of orientation, discussed in Chapter XXXII. Particular attention should be paid to those areas where the applicant, if approved, would work.

EMPLOYEE HANDBOOK. An employee handbook either should be given to the applicant for review at his leisure, or can be given to him for study while in the facility. The former approach is considered best, providing enough are available.

By following these steps you are ensured to a significant degree that the employee you hire is actually matched to the job involved. And even if you decide against hiring him, you have explained something about nursing homes in general and your nursing home in particular and, hopefully, through intelligent and courteous handling of the matter, possibly have created a friend.

Former Employees

This section possibly should be retitled "About To Be Former Employees," as it concerns those employees who have decided to stop working for you. In the case of amicable partings, where the employee is leaving for personal reasons or similar, it is advised to maintain contact, continue the person on the mailing list for your newsletter, and invite him to appropriate functions. In this manner you keep close contact with those who can perhaps help when you are in dire need, or when you least expect it.

In cases where the leave-taking is not so amicable, where the person leaving clearly is dissatisfied for one reason or another, we strongly recommend an exit interview which will help determine what went wrong. The information gained from such an interview can be very important for, to an extent, it probably is the hiring mechanism which failed, not getting the right person in the first place. Additionally, it may point out some problems with personnel or policies which you never realized existed. A frank talk is the best kind, and you should be encouraged to draw out the truth if at all possible. Emphasize that your reasons for knowing are based upon a desire to improve the situation so it will not happen again. In some cases it could mean giving the employee a chance to blow off steam and hence turn a potential enemy into someone who is at least neutral. There may also be the situation which will enable you to take immediate corrective action, and perhaps keep the employee on through mutual consent.

XXXIII

VOLUNTEER RELATIONS

HUNDREDS OF THOUSANDS of words have been written on the benefits of a nursing home volunteer program. The most immediately perceived benefits accrue to patients. Even friendly visitors form a link with the community at large, and their genuine interest in patient well-being without any economic motivation is a significant morale booster for those who often regard themselves as forgotten by the world about them.

From a less idealistic point of view, a volunteer program is a service taken into serious consideration by those selecting a nursing home for themselves or others, and the volunteer public offers management a very powerful tool in overall PR programing.

Volunteer Program as a PR Tool

Considering the volunteer program from the aspect of a PR tool, it first is necessary to understand the public involved. Typically, those who volunteer are activists in the community usually involved in a variety of worthwhile endeavors. As such, they are leaders, and their opinions and observations usually are held in high regard by others. Obviously, what they think about your nursing home has weight regardless of circumstances, but is even more highly respected when it is understood that their opinions are based on firsthand experience.

For the most part, what volunteers think of your nursing home will be dependent on what your nursing home really is like. If you want volunteers to tell others that every effort is made to care for patients well; that management and staff really are concerned about patient welfare, then, in fact, every effort must be made to care for patients well and demonstrate real concern for their welfare. If all possible efforts in this direction are not expended, volunteers will be quick to realize it, and the image developed will simply reflect conditions as they are. Any attempts

143

to falsify image-forming factors will only worsen the situation; will lower credibility of management in volunteers' eyes, and become incorporated into an unflattering, though somewhat accurate image.

Therefore, the primary concern with the volunteer public is commitment: Commitment to the best patient care possible, and commitment to honesty and openness in management/volunteer relations.

Other concerns, especially those involving communication, require recognition of the volunteer's status within the nursing home. A volunteer is, by definition, unpaid, but the positive feeling obtained from being of meaningful assistance provides what is called psychic income. Recognition of value and increased opportunities to be of value increase psychic income and, accordingly, are appreciated. Conversely, lack of recognition and appreciation or limitation of opportunities is resented. Also, while volunteers are part of the nursing home family, their primary allegiance is to patients. They owe management nothing. What respect management hopes to attain must be earned.

Management Factors

While this chapter is not intended to tell you how to establish or run your program—there are many other materials available on this subject—certain management points should be emphasized for their importance to effective volunteer relations.

ORGANIZATION. For the program to function well it must be managed well. This means that the various materials available should be studied thoroughly and modified as necessary to meet the unique circumstances of your nursing home.

DIRECTOR. The program must have a paid, trained director, either a staff member with dual responsibilities or a person whose sole work is volunteer program director. A trained director can assure maximum effectiveness of volunteer efforts through careful management and scheduling. Further, a paid director owes a certain amount of allegiance to management, and therefore can provide excellent liaison and a communications conduit between management and volunteers.

VOLUNTEER ORIENTATION. As with employees, the methods used to bring volunteers into the program can have great bearing on ultimate performance. Volunteers must be informed of appropriate dos and don'ts, each supplemented with a "why"; must be told frankly of some of the problems they can expect, especially in regard to patient personalities; should be informed of management's patient care goals, and the accompanying restrictions and limitations. More specifically, volunteers must be made to understand that some patients will scheme to play upon their emotions and that others, perhaps nasty and argumentative in their younger years, have found no reason to change their ways in later years.

EMPLOYEE ORIENTATION. It is especially critical that employees are oriented toward volunteers in an effective manner. This requires telling key staff members, or all employees if possible, that volunteers will need assistance, and that their efforts deserve employee support and patience. It should be emphasized that volunteers will be telling others of their experiences and observations and employees will be responsible to a very great extent for what volunteers think of the facility. In fact, by emphasizing this latter point, you will stress the importance of staff within the nursing home community and so minimize some of the resentment and jealousy which volunteers can sometimes engender within the ranks of employees.

Tools for Effective Volunteer Relations

Obviously, the more effective volunteer relations become, the more volunteers feel as though they are a part of the nursing home, and the more allegiance they feel to the home itself, over and above that which they feel toward patients. Establishment of such effective relations requires recognition of the unique status of volunteers, and incorporation of the entire program into the fabric of overall activities.

In this light, many of the tools and programs utilized for other publics apply here, such as:

INDUCE RECOGNITION. Volunteers should be recognized as individuals through use of press releases, bulletin board items, volunteer of the month features, name badges, knowledge of name by management, and similar factors.

ACCOMPLISHMENT RECOGNITION. Recognition of volunteers' accomplishments is especially important in light of the volunteer's need for psychic income. Such recognition can be developed through personal talks, articles in the newsletter, development of "good news" stories in the local press, awards (including pins indicating hours volunteered), increased responsibilities, and similar activities.

SELF-GOVERNMENT. Providing volunteers with an element of self-government, coordinated with overall rules and regulations, particularly takes volunteers unique status into consideration. A volunteers' council, for example, working in conjunction with management, allows new programs and policies to be developed in light of firsthand experience. Moreover, it demonstrates management's willingness to give volunteers and the volunteer program a degree of autonony when it is felt to be in the best interest of patients.

GENERAL INVOLVEMENT. The extent to which volunteers are allowed to participate in general programs, many of which are established for employees, should be the result of careful consideration of the individual circumstances within your nursing home. If employee relations are not as good as you would like them to be, volunteer involvement in certain employee programs could limit their employee-directed goals. Perhaps the most effective strategy is to work through an employees council to determine staff attitudes and feelings, leaving the choice up to them. Conversely, volunteers may elect to establish their own, parallel programs, a decision to be made by the volunteers' council.

SPECIFIC PROGRAMS/CONCERNS. There are some elements of an overall volunteer relations program that deserve specific mention and consideration:

UNIFORMS. If your volunteer program consists of little more than friendly visiting, uniforms are not necessary, although name badges would be advisable. If volunteers are active in other aspects, however, as in an activities program, uniforms, distinct from employees', are desirable. It is not necessary for management to furnish uniforms, but it is an appreciated gesture, especially when proprietary facilities are involved.

HOUR BADGES. Management should award volunteers with hour badges indicating the amount of hours volunteered, such as 250, 500, etc. It recognizes volunteer efforts; creates a bond between nursing home and individual volunteers, and gives the volunteer an incentive to volunteer even additional time. Presentation of such awards and others discussed below, should be somewhat ceremonious to add meaning to the award itself. Having patients presenting the award is particularly meaningful.

CERTIFICATES. Appropriate certificates, framed or suitable for framing, can be presented after a volunteer completes training; in recognition of one year's activity or giving of a certain amount of hours per year, or in recognition of other achievements. You can have such certificates printed easily, but they should be printed well.

BANQUET. Volunteers and perhaps spouses, could be treated to an annual banquet by management. In cases of awards presentation, know in advance (as to the volunteer putting in the most hours) , family would be on hand.

Also, many other items included throughout the book and especially relating to employee relations can be applied for effective relations with the volunteer community.

XXXIV

COMMUNITY (GROUP)
RELATIONS

PERHAPS THE MOST effective way to establish direct relations with the community is to establish direct relations with various community groups. In addition to speaking before such groups, you should strive to establish meaningful, continuing contact especially on behalf of patients. Garden clubs could be encouraged to work with patients in planting; the Red Cross probably can involve patients in various volunteer activities; involvement with political organizations can turn the nursing home into a beehive of activity, and so on. To an extent, much of this type work can be undertaken in the context of an activities program, which should be acutely aware of community resources.

Community groups of all types also should be given the opportunity to utilize your facilities, if possible. Various organizations frequently need a place to meet and, by being of assistance, the nursing home can become regarded as a group resource. Further, such contacts afford opportunities for additional contact, which in turn helps foster understanding of nursing homes in general, and your home in particular.

Community group interaction also can come about through open house activities, interesting guest speakers, movies, and similar events, as well as through participation of key staff members in various organizations, involving themselves and the nursing home as appropriate.

In all dealings with community groups, bear in mind that the more person-to-person contact there is, the more understanding there is. By interacting with many community groups, the nursing home itself becomes an acknowledged community resource, a status whose positive benefits cannot be overemphasized.

XXXV

HEALTH CARE
PUBLIC RELATIONS

T HE HEALTH CARE public, which deserves attention, includes the
entire local health care public, as well as certain elements of
state and health care publics.

Local

Locally, an effort should be made to determine which institutions and organizations are involved in health care, including
hospitals, clinics, other nursing homes, day care centers, associations of professional and paraprofessional personnel, and so forth.
The list can be supplemented by names of certain key individuals.
By knowing who comprises the public involved, you have at least
a tool to be used if and when it is necessary, as well as a tool which
permits continuing contact. As an example, the list can be developed as a mailing list for sending of newsletters, press releases
and other materials.

It is strongly suggested that interaction be more than just communications. For example, you could conduct an open house for
a group of health professionals; offer the home as a training area
for student nurses, medical students, and others; work with others
in establishment and/or implementation of a community health
care organization, in general becoming involved to as great an
extent as practically possible. By becoming so involved, your interest and abilities become recognized, and you and your nursing
home are able to assume a deserved place of prominence in your
community's overall health care system. It possibly could lead to
the establishment of additional services which your nursing home
could offer in response to observed needs, such as a day care
center, meals on wheels, and so forth.

State

On the state level, participation in affairs of the health care community can be developed through membership in various associations of administrators, nurses, and others. Service on various committees should be encouraged to foster comprehensive knowledge of current developments, and to ensure recognition of the nursing home's point of view in establishment of association positions and attitudes. Naturally, sufficient time off should be given to those personnel who participate in association activities.

National

Nationally, activity should be devoted at least to nursing home affairs through participation in organizations such as ANHA, AAHA, ACNHA, and others. Such participation broadens knowledge of the overall involvement of nursing homes within the health care industry, much of which is usable on the local level.

XXXVI

GOVERNMENT OFFICIAL RELATIONS

I T IS NO secret that virtually every nursing home in the United States must each day contend with an amazing variety of federal, state and local laws and regulations. Behind each law and regulation is a government agency entrusted with its implementation. And within each agency is an individual or two who will have direct interaction with your nursing home.

Naturally, what a government official is most interested in is compliance with the law or regulation it is his duty to enforce. At issue is your home's compliance, in most cases a matter of cut-and-dried statistics. Ostensibly, whether the government official involved likes you, dislikes you or doesn't know you from Adam has little bearing. But the facts of the matter are that we all are human beings and enjoy being treated as such. If establishment of good relations with government officials, which involves little more than establishment of good communications, means that you will on occasion get the benefit of the doubt, then clearly it's worth the effort. In truth, however, establishment of good relations may mean far more than occasional benefits in cases of legally authorized discretion. Government officials are involved in your industry and your profession. They can and should be called upon for assistance when it's needed, just as they should be able to call upon you for guidance, perhaps to assist in development of new, more responsible regulations, or to serve as an instructor in a government-sponsored course. As with any public, the goal should be establishment of mutual understanding and good will so that if and when one ever needs the other, assistance can be expected. If nothing is done to foster good relations, then little can be done at the last minute when an unexpected crisis occurs.

Who

The first step in establishing good relations with any public is to know who the public is. In the case of government officials, you should have on file the name, address and telephone number of each appropriate national, regional, state, and local government agency; the names of directors, and names of staff members with whom you work. Most information can be compiled by using a telephone, local offices usually having state, regional or national information at hand.

Communicate

Once you determine who the public is, the next step is to communicate with its members. Consider writing a letter to each department or agency head involved (individually or robo typed) stating your intentions to communicate via sending your home's newsletter, press releases and similar periodic issuances. You also may wish to include other material such as a brochure, employees' manual, patients' handbook, etc., asking, where appropriate, for comments or suggestions for improvements. In the same letter ask for reciprocal consideration from the department or agency involved. Should you not have a newsletter, brochure or similar material, a letter simply asking for department or agency publications is not inappropriate.

In cases of officials with whom you come into frequent contact, more personalized communications also are acceptable, such as Christmas cards on birthday greetings.

Activities

Officials can be invited to certain key activities held during the year, including special banquets, patient art shows, and others which relate primarily to and illustrate patient care and nursing home patient interaction.

Official Business

When an official is in the home on official business every effort should be made to provide assistance. Pertinent materials should be readily accessible and those with answers to questions should be on hand.

Association Matters

Frequently a state nursing home association, or related group, will feature a guest speaker whom certain officials may find interesting. Be certain to inform them (even if the association probably already has informed him) and, if feasible, offer a ride.

XXXVII

NEWS MEDIA RELATIONS

METHODS OF CONTACTING the news media are mentioned throughout this book, ranging from issuance of news releases to telephone calls, requests for assistance in developing an in-house newsletter, and so forth. If you have done little with the news media public, however, the following should be considered.

Let news media representatives know who you are and let them know you're around. By all means, write a letter to all area editors, including broadcast news assignment editors, indicating that you will be undertaking a program of increased community involvement. Ask for their consideration, and offer assistance in matters of health care, problems of aging, and related subjects. A typical letter would be as follows:

```
Mr. John Smith
Health Editor
Anytown Tribune

Dear Mr. Smith:

This is to inform you that XYZ Nursing Home
shortly will begin a program of increased
community involvement primarily for our
patients whose health and well-being can be
improved through evidence of community
concern. We will be attempting to inform you
of what we are doing through issuance of news
releases and personal calls, and we hope you
find some of our activities worthy of coverage.
In the meantime, should you ever require source
persons for stories relating to long-term care,
nursing home issues, problems of aging, or
related items, we will be happy to be of
service to the best of our ability.
```

154

We look forward to working with you, and hope
to be of service in the future.

Sincerely,

Continued communication should be undertaken through issuance of news releases (and occasional letters of thanks for extensive coverage) ; visits to meet the news media representative in person; issuing to news media representatives copies of your newsletter, as well as special materials which may be available from your nursing home association, such as facts fillers, fact books and related materials.

Bear in mind that the news media public represents a conduit public through which many others are reached. By maintaining contact; by trying to be of genuine service; by being frank and candid, you can develop effective relationships which will enable more accurate reporting, and greater realization of the problems with which you must contend.

INDEX